Fibromyalgia and Chronic Fatigue

Acutherapy and Holistic Approaches

A Guide for Holistic Practitioners and the People they Work With

Sunny Cooper, M.S., O.B.T.

Life Circles Publications
965 East 28th Street
Ogden UT 84403

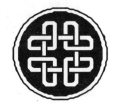

First Edition: January 1, 2000 A.D.
Printed and Bound in the United States of America

ISBN 0-9674577-0-X

LCCN 99-066573

ATTENTION ORGANIZATIONS, SCHOOLS OF HEALING ARTS, AND THERAPY CLINICS AND CENTERS: Quantity discounts are available on bulk purchases of this book for educational purposes or fund raising. For information please contact the publisher.

Published by Life Circles Publications
965 East 28th Street
Ogden UT 84403
Phone (801)-612-1306

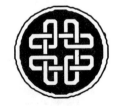

TABLE OF CONTENTS

Preface and Acknowledgements

I first heard the term "fibromyalgia" in 1994 when I attended a symposium on the subject in Baton Rouge, Louisiana, where I lived at the time. I had been practicing oriental bodywork for about seven years, and had clients from time to time who claimed they hurt all over and did not know what was wrong with them in spite of numerous visits to doctors and many dollars spent on diagnostic tests. The symposium was led by Richard Vanwhy, a scholar, researcher, and author on fibromyalgia, and was sponsored by our state chapter of the American Massage Therapy Association. Attending were massage and bodywork practitioners and a handful of people who had fibromyalgia. Everyone got to tell their stories.

This symposium was the beginning of a new phase of my personal and professional journey. As all the people were telling their stories and sharing information, I listened and took lots of notes, organizing what was said by the models of traditional Chinese medicine which I had been working with. All the different symptoms that were reported seemed to fit neatly into several of the common patterns of disharmony that acutherapists and herbalists work with: Stagnation of Liver Qi, Deficiency of Spleen Qi, and presence of the Damp pathogen seemed to account for most of the symptoms reported by the people in attendance.

Shortly after that I began to see numerous individuals in my practice who had fibromyalgia and chronic fatigue. Even some of the students in the shiatsu classes I was teaching had one or the other or both of these syndromes. It seemed that I had found my way into what I have come to call an "energy vortex" containing the disharmonies called fibromyalgia and chronic fatigue. Everyone intuitively knows what energy vortexes are, especially practitioners who seem to attract a certain kind of client into their clinic. Some practitioners seem to work with lots of cancer patients; others draw the AIDS community to their workspace, for me it is the fibromyalgia and chronic fatigue clients.

I believe each type of illness has come into our collective lives bringing certain opportunities to learn. All the people who are learning that particular lesson tend to travel together for awhile, some as clients, some as practitioners, some as writers or teachers or researchers on the subject. Energy vortices are archetypal patterns that "suck in" the people who resonate with that pattern, and we do this in groups, sharing many kinds of experiences including health challenges, with others in that vortex. Right next to us are people having different kinds of experiences, and even though we may pass them on the street or in the workplace every day, we just never seem to quite connect. They are in their vortex, and we are in ours.

For the next eighteen months almost everybody I worked with had fibromyalgia or chronic fatigue or both. I learned alot, and got to test my ideas about oriental medical therapy for these people. Pretty soon other bodywork practitioners started to ask me what I was doing, because my clients were gradually getting better. In 1995 I wrote a sixty-page monograph entitled "Oriental Bodywork and Fibromyalgia Syndrome". This was mainly for massage and bodywork practitioners and their clients. Four years later I have learned so much more that I want to share, and offer this to other types of practitioners and their clients as well. This book replaces the earlier one, and it was renamed in an attempt to capture the wider scope.

So what have fibromyalgia and chronic fatigue come to teach us? Until the late 1980's nobody really knew much about them even though they are cited in medical literature for the entire century. It was only in 1990 that the American College of Rheumatology defined the criteria for physicians to use when diagnosing fibromyalgia. Still, as of this writing, a hefty number of physicians do not believe these are "real" illnesses.

Many diseases which were dominant prior to World War II hardly exist any more, at least in the US and other technological countries. Diphtheria, typhus, yellow fever, plague, malaria, small pox, dysentery and other infectious diseases were the big killers. Infection of wounds goes in this category also. There was a time when the mention of these diseases brought as much terror as cancer and AIDS do today. What were the learnings brought to our culture by these diseases? We learned about sanitation, infectious agents, and medical practitioners learned how to practice sterile examinations and interventions to avoid spreading infectious agents among their patients. Antibiotics were developed. These learnings profoundly altered the way we live in terms of sanitation and personal hygiene. In modern cultures every household has at least one toilet, drinking water and waste water are kept separate, sewage processing has evolved, and many other changes have arisen out of the experience of overcoming those diseases.

Meanwhile there was another group of infectious diseases such as polio, influenza, and measles. These are not usually transmitted by contaminated water or surgeon's instruments or insect vectors. They are airborne or transmitted by contact with infected individuals or their body fluids. Another type of disease brought another type of problem to solve, and another advance in health care came from this group: vaccines. Vaccination has become a mainstay of medical practice since the 1940's. A large amount of money still goes into developing vaccines which will protect people from AIDS and other diseases.

Now we have the new echelon of "functional disease". Fibromyalgia, chronic fatigue and chronic pain syndromes, along with a host of other autoimmnune disorders and stress related illnesses have become major health concerns in the last thirty years. These are gaining in prevalence and probably now comprise the bulk of a primary care physician's practice. So what have they come to teach us?

We have come to where we now stand in health care through the door of "medicine". I mean this quite literally. Drugs, medications, pharmaceuticals, pills, whatever one chooses to call them, these have been the basis of treating diseases for most of the twentieth century. This trend started with the availability of sulpha drugs in the 1930's and has formed the foundation of health care ever since.

This new generation of chronic illness is difficult to treat with drugs. At best, people try to "manage" their chronic illness. No new "miracle cures" have shown up for a very long time. So what are we, personally and collectively, to learn from this? I believe we are now in the midst of an opportunity to learn personal responsibility for our actions and their consequences, including the health consequences. Our actions include our behaviors, our lifestyle choices, our emotional responses, our spiritual practices, and the ways we take care of our physical bodies. Consequences include emotional imbalances such as depression, chronic stress and physical illness. Related to these are problems in relationships, dissatisfaction with our jobs and careers, and feeling of lonely and detached from meaningful experiences.

Fibromyalgia and chronic fatigue are exquisite examples of disharmonies in which the client is the key determinant of improvement. There is no single approach or therapy or practice which reverses these disharmonies. Nobody can "fix" a person who has these disharmonies, or take away their illness. Each person must develop his or her own healing path. These two syndromes challenge the person to re-evaluate lifestyle choices, relationships, belief system, and self-concept. Illness is an invitation to transformation; those who accept the invitation and show up for the party tend to do very well in their recovery, and this often leads to personal evolution of a kind they never would have achieved without the challenge of chronic pain and fatigue.

This is a book for people who want to empower themselves and recover from these illnesses through holistic therapies and personal transformation. It is also for holistically oriented practitioners who work with them: acupuncturists, oriental bodywork therapists, massage therapists, chiropractors, naturopaths, herbalists, holistic nutrition counsellors, hypnotherapists, mental health counsellors, nurses, and physicians.

The concepts of the holistic paradigm have been in existence for thousands of years. I find it interesting that the parts of the world where they developed are presently second- and third- world nations. These cultures are now strongly attracted to bring modern mainstream medicine to their people while we are beginning to incorporate age-old concepts into our medical system. We are circling in each other's footsteps as we move toward a way of integrating the best of mainstream medicine with the heart and soul of healing which lies within each one of us.

Throughout this book I have used the term "client" to denote the individual who is seeking assistance from a "practitioner" or "therapist." I have consciously chosen to avoid the word "patient" except in the context of medical research or treatment. These words connote a particular type of relationship between two people, one as helper and one seeking help. The word "patient" refers to an individual seeking assistance from a medical or surgical doctor. In some of the United States verbiage has legal connotations; for example a massage therapist cannot "diagnose" or "treat". They must call what they do "assessment" and "balancing" or some such paraphrasing. Likewise, holistic practitioners have a different relationship with the people who come to them, and that relationship deserves a different word to describe it. I have chosen the word "client" to characterize this relationship. I have also chosen to use primarily feminine pronouns (her, she) because the strong majority of those with fibromyalgia and chronic fatigue are women. In some cases I have used masculine pronouns, or mixed gender (his/her) when concepts apply in a more general sense to people of both genders.

This book has chapters on topics which I have not seen in the popular books on fibromyalgia and chronic fatigue: body-mind concepts of pain management; lymphatic work; rebuilding the immune system, and a discussion of the holistic paradigm and personal characteristics which contribute to health or illness. I hope this will contribute to the learning and evolution of all who read it.

I wish to express gratitude to some of the people who have accompanied me or facilitated my journey: Vernon Smith (my shiatsu teacher); Regina Drueding MD (my friend and fellow traveller); all the clients and students who have shared experiences with me, and my mate Homer who has graciously tolerated all my obsessiveness over the years. Some of the teachers who have changed my life (in approximately chronological order) include Vernon Smith, Ned Holle, Orisia Haas, Benny Vaughn, Cindy Banker, Kiiko Matsumoto, Richard Bandler, Rick Gold, Joseph Thomas, Bill Helm and Arnie Lade. Special thanks to Vernon Smith, Arnie Lade, and Devorah Segall for the precious time they each spent reviewing the manuscript and offering many valuable suggestions for this project.

TABLES

DIAGRAMS

APPENDICES

Chapter 1

Introduction to Fibromyalgia and Chronic Fatigue

Fibromyalgia Syndrome (FMS) and Chronic Fatigue Immune Deficiency Syndrome (CFIDS) are complex disorders involving a variety of symptom patterns. They are classified as "syndromes" because they do not meet the criteria to be classified as "diseases". To be classified as a disease, there must be 1) known cause, 2) well understood pathology, and 3) a set of signs and symptoms which occurs in each individual with the disease. Fibromyalgia and chronic fatigue syndromes meet none of these criteria.

These two syndromes are more prevalent in women than men (approximately 90% are women), and can occur in young children and teens. The prevalence of fibromyalgia syndrome in the general population has been estimated to be 2%, with incidence increasing with age; the prevalence of CFIDS is much less than that of FMS (Goldenberg, 1996). The two syndromes bear two separate names but seem to co-exist in many people, and are probably two different presentations of the same underlying process. For the purposes of discussion in this text we will assume that this is an accurate statement. For the individuals who live with these syndromes, and for the holistic physicians and practitioners who work with them, the technical distinction, if any, is less important than many other factors.

While there are several common elements in the presentation of all FMS and CFIDS clients, there is also variation in the types and severity of symptoms. Individual response to therapeutic interventions and impact on the client's ability to function effectively varies widely. The adverse impact on quality of life is probably more dramatic than most health care professionals have recognized (Burckhard, et al. 1993).

The term "fibromyalgia" has appeared in the medical literature for approximately ninety years, yet it may still go unrecognized and undiagnosed by physicians. It is probably more common than rheumatoid arthritis, and yet it's medical cause, if any, remains unknown. (Cunningham, 1996) There is no known medical cause or medical cure, and medical treatments are aimed at reducing symptoms and managing one's condition. Other terms have been used to describe this condition including "fibrositis", "muscular rheumatism", "myofibrositis", and "myodysneuria" (Vanwhy, 1997). In Great Britain, Myalgic Encephalitis (ME) is the term used for both fibromyalgia and chronic fatigue syndromes.

Fibromyalgia is considered chronic, non-inflammatory, systemic, and non-degenerative; no structural damage is attributed to it, as, for example, in degenerative disk disease, where the disks lose structural integrity over time. People with fibromyalgia and chronic fatigue can, however, improve over time and many actually go into remission, with symptoms being minimal and having little interference with their health and comfort. In a ten year follow-up study of fibromyalgia patients who had an average duration of symptoms of 15.8 years, researchers found that all the patients still had symptoms. These included moderate to severe pain or stiffness in 55% of the subjects, moderate to extreme sleep difficulty in 48%, and moderate to extreme fatigue in 59%. Most reported some improvement of symptoms over the course of their illness (Kennedy and Felson, 1996).

Asian-based physiotherapy (Oriental bodywork, acupuncture, exercise), lifestyle modification, and personal growth are key strategies for moving toward recovery. Much will be said about these concepts throughout this book. Many people with chronic fatigue or fibromyalgia have been able to make vast improvements in their condition using the methods in this book.

ONSET OF FIBROMYALGIA AND CHRONIC FATIGUE

Numerous physiological imbalances are seen in fibromyalgia and chronic fatigue clients, including nutritional deficiencies, acquired toxicity, inadequate stress coping abilities, sensitivities and allergies, inappropriate or excessive medication, blood sugar imbalance, hormonal imbalance, poor posture and breathing, immune challenges from current or past infections, impaired organs of digestion and elimination, and emotional distress. It is unclear whether any of these are in a direct causal relationship with the onset or whether they stem from a shared cause.

Onset of fibromyalgia and chronic fatigue can be sudden or gradual. There is a recurring theme of three factors among fibromyalgia clients. We will consider each of these factors in turn. The three are:

1) High-stress lifestyle
2) Weakened immune system, and
3) Emotional or physical trauma.

High Stress Lifestyles

High stress lifestyles are almost ubiquitous in the United States and other developed countries. Our modern culture has traded the stresses of survival found in third-world nations for a whole system of new stresses which arise out of the technology and information-based society.

Only since the 1970's have Western-trained physicians seriously considered the role of diet, stress, mental patterns and emotions as causes of illness. There is still, however, much resistance to these ideas. In the New England Journal of Medicine in 1985, an editorial by NEJM Deputy Editor Dr. Marcia Nygell, announced that "It is time to acknowledge that our belief in disease as a direct reflection of mental state is largely folklore". Even as recently as 1990, a survey of MD's taken by the American Medical Association concluded that 90% of those responding did not see mental or emotional causes as being related to disease process. However, much of the current "wellness movement" centers around behavioral aspects of disease prevention by teaching stress management techniques, body awareness, self care, family support, physical conditioning, and cognitive training.

According to traditional Chinese medicine (TCM), there are several major causes of disharmony and disease. Interestingly, these are mostly related to stressful living which arises when one fails to live "according to the natural laws." The "natural laws" describe a lifestyle which features moderation of all things, a balanced way of living, reverence and respect for nature, and a path of spiritual development leading to self-mastery. (See Appendix 3). This is quite different from the Western view of the cause of disease from invading pathogens or failure of organs.

For the practitioner of traditional Chinese medicine these things are signs of advanced, unattended problems which started years previously. They may be treated with herbs or bodywork or needles, but if the client is to have any hope of recovering, they must return to "living according to the natural laws." It was years of unbalanced living which weakened them enough to be vulnerable to pathogens or organ failure. Chinese doctors equate going for treatment after illness has begun to "digging a well after one is already feeling thirst" and "forging weapons as the enemy is burning the village. Some of the more common types of stress will be explored as they relate to fibromyalgia and chronic fatigue.

These patterns of stress, when prolonged, typically lead to conditions of "running on empty" and "burn out". Poor nutrition, sedentary indoor lifestyles, lack of appropriate movement, insufficient sleep, and lack of emotional support increase the amount of "burn out" a person experiences. This condition of chronic "burn out" or "running on empty" is virtually universal in individuals who develop fibromyalgia. It is important for the practitioner to remember that all disharmony or disease is the result of multiple causes, and there are many combinations of stressors which could be relevant for a particular individual with fibromyalgia or chronic fatigue.

Often the most significant improvements come not from therapeutic intervention, but from the person's own choices and lifestyle changes. The prognosis for FMS and CFIDS is unpredictable; some studies show remission in almost one quarter of cases and improvement in almost one half of cases two years after diagnosis (Granges, Zilko, and Littlejohn, 1994). Other studies confirm poor outcomes with marked functional disability and emotional effects four years after diagnosis (Ledingham, et al, 1993).

Family stress:

Evolving societal trends have led to numerous alternative lifestyles, including single parent families resulting from divorce, single parent families resulting from choice not to have a partner, gay and lesbian couples, gay and lesbian couples raising children, couples living in different cities for job or other reasons, families with step-children and step-parents as a result of second or third marriages, non-custodial parents living apart from the children yet obligated to provided financial support, unmarried childless individuals living alone, and geographical separation from grandparents and other close relatives. Each of these situations generates different stresses in terms of societal expectations, task allocation, role identification, distribution of time and financial resources, disputes over child-rearing decisions, unresolved emotional issues, and many other factors. Family stresses are likely to continue for extended periods of time and become an everyday factor in the fabric of peoples' lives. Often individuals lose sight of the degree to which these factors can drain their energy and affect their health.

Occupational stress

Jobs and school are a source of stress for many people. Familiar examples include conflicts with bosses or co-workers, time spent commuting to work, performance stress, deadlines, overtime, shift work, distractions and interruptions, down-sizing and other organizational changes in companies, fear of losing one's job or being transferred, union activities, conflict between job and personal or family demands, and salary and benefit concerns. In addition to these, many people have high degrees of exposure to computer monitors, fluorescent lighting, synthetic building materials, and chemicals used in the job place. Others stresses include sedentary desk jobs, and repetitive motion injuries at computers and other types of jobs. It is rare to find an individual who thoroughly enjoys his/her job and finds it contributes positively to health.

In Chinese medical theory over-work is regarded as a common source of disharmony (Maciocia, 1989). Over-work may be physical or mental. Too much thinking or studying without resting can be just as injurious as too much physical labor. The amount of work must also be paced to the individual's condition. Weak, old, or infirm people have lower tolerance for mental or physical work than those who are strong, young, and healthy. Too much work damages both the Yin and Yang of the body. Problems may come soon after excessive laboring, or the results may accumulate over time.

Nutritional Stress

The typical American diet, with frequent consumption of meat, fat, and sugar, causes the body a great deal of stress. Lack of nutrients and excesses of chemicals and toxins contribute to poor physiological functioning, chemical imbalances, and tissue breakdown. Other factors which contribute to nutritional stress are irregular meal times and conditions of eating. Eating while working, while emotionally upset, over-tired, or otherwise stressed can interfere with smooth digestion and utilization of food. Over- or under-eating, chaotic eating, eating late at night, and skipping breakfast also create disharmony in the digestive process.

The Chinese medical approach to diet is different than the food-groups, food-pyramids, macro- and micro-nutrients of modern western nutrition (Haas, 1981; Lu, 1986). Oriental nutrition considers the relationship between the person and the food he consumes. Poor diet can indeed arise from inadequate quality or quantity of food, but another element in the equation is "who is eating the food". Many people who eat high quality food still suffer from nutritional problems if they are not able to effectively digest, absorb, distribute, and utilize the food, or if the food is not appropriate to their condition.

Oriental nutrition emphasizes the energetic quality of foods more than the biochemical constituents of the food. Some foods create a warming, tonifying, strengthening, tightening, or contracting (Yang) effect on the body. Others cause cooling, calming, dispersing, sedating, weakening, loosening, or expanding (Yin) effect on the body. A diet may be well-balanced according to Western nutrients and food-groups, and still be too Yin or too

Yang for a person's condition. When this is the case a person may think his diet is appropriate, and therefore completely overlook the benefits of dietary changes which may help chronic patterns such as fibromyalgia and chronic fatigue. Working with foods is a powerful therapeutic modality for people with chronic conditions (Pitchford, 1993).

Technological stress

Technological stress comes in many forms including the processing of foods, appliances and personal electronic devices, transportation, use of pesticides and herbicides, and computer technology. In some ways technology makes our lives easier, it also seems to make things more complicated and challenging for many.

Information stress

Computers and the internet have added to the mountains of information people are exposed to and must process. This includes the huge amounts of printed material which arrive in our mailboxes every day, advertising, television programming, books and magazines, newspapers and Email.

Information overload can quickly become overwhelming. A person with a few financial investments may have hours of reading to do each month to make decisions about his investments. Professional people are deluged with information concerning their fields of expertise. People are turning to information sources to solve a myriad of problems from the challenges of child-rearing to retraining for a new career, to learning how to get through the changes in their lives with a minimum of damage. Information is here to stay, but we are still in the process of figuring out how to screen, sort, process, interpret, save, update, and delete information, in a way that relieves stress instead of adding to it.

Iatrogenic stress

Going to the doctor has always been a stressful event for many people, and this is increasingly a factor which can influence one's health in a negative way. The practice of medicine has become much more de-personalized with the advent of "managed care". Yet the number of drugs available, both prescription and over-the-counter, keeps increasing, and all can potentially have serious side effects, especially with long-term usage. Adverse reactions to prescription drugs are estimated to be the sixth leading cause of death in the US in hospitalized patients, and many more people suffer from side effects (Lazarou et al, 1998).

The mainstream medical system has further removed the individual from the formula of treatment, diluting the person's authority in his own life and promoting dependence on the medical practitioner. Meanwhile, physicians frequently have their hands tied by insurance guidelines and cannot always do as much for a patient as they might otherwise. While advances in medical technology have seemingly produced miracles, there is a high price to pay in terms of stress for both practitioners and patients.

Many people with chronic illness such as fibromyalgia and chronic fatigue tend to "doc-hop", going to specialist after specialist, trying different drugs, looking for a magic bullet that can "cure" their problems. They are inevitably met with failure as new symptoms arise and their overall health gradually declines. They are looking for an external cause and an external cure for their misery instead of looking inward. This can lead to high levels of stress, both from the interventions that are employed, and from the disappointment and failure that occurs repeatedly. In itself, turning over one's personal authority to external people or situations is a key component in stress (see Chapter 3)

Financial stress

Most people in our culture experience intermittent financial stress, and many experience it chronically. Spending habits, societal and personal pressure for acquiring material goods, easy access to credit cards and loans contribute to this stress. In the context of health, many people claim they "can't afford" products and therapies which may increase their well-being and improve their health problems. Dependence on third party providers is common in our culture, and many individuals categorically rule out any type of treatment which their insurance doesn't cover, even when they could afford to pay out-of-pocket. Oriental bodywork, acupuncture, herbs, massage therapy, and many other excellent complementary modalities are rarely covered by typical health insurance.

Weakened Immune System

When stress is uninterrupted and prolonged, the immune system will eventually become weakened. The physiology of stress has been described in many texts on stress and stress management (Seaward, 1994). The immune system may also be weakened by acute illness such as colds and flu. Many cases of fibromyalgia and chronic fatigue seem to start with an acute viral illness which never resolves completely.

Signals of immune suppression can include:

1. Fatigue
2. Catches colds or flu easily, and illness persists for a long time
3. Allergies worsen
4. Low stress tolerance
5. Hormonal imbalances, including thyroid and female hormone problems
6. Chronic or recurring infections, such as sinus, vaginal, throat, systemic yeast (Candida), or herpesvirus (genital, cold sores, and shingles) coupled with history of frequent use of antibiotics
7. Slow wound healing and easy bruising
8. Easily chilled, feeling of being "cold in the bones". Seriously immune-suppressed individuals usually dislike winter and cold weather.

Rebuilding the immune system is a key strategy in optimizing one's probability of improvement or recovery from fibromyalgia and chronic fatigue. This will be the subject of Chapter 8.

Physical or Emotional Trauma

Physical Trauma

Past physical trauma is almost universally a part of the history of fibromyalgia clients. Examples of trauma may include falls, motor vehicle accidents, sports injuries, and surgical operations. Major dental work such as root canals or extractions, and prolonged labor and difficult delivery are also traumatic to the body. Spinal injury, bone fractures, head trauma, loss of blood, and internal injury are also traumas to the body.

Multiple traumatic experiences, including sexual and physical abuse may be important initiating factors (Goldenberg, 1996). Another report (Taylor, et al, 1995) concluded that sexual abuse does not appear to be a specific factor in the etiology of FMS, but is correlated with the number and severity of associated symptoms. Many fibromyalgia clients have had multiple traumas, some of which may have occurred years before the onset of the syndrome. In some cases onset is sudden following an accident or surgery. This sudden onset has been referred to as "reactive" fibromyalgia and was found to be the case in 23% of patients in one study (Greenfield, et al, 1992).

Multiple abdominal surgeries are common in the histories fibromyalgia clients. Appendectomy, gall bladder surgery, and hernia repairs are quite common abdominal procedures. Multiple abdominal surgeries are commonly seen in women who have had Caesarean deliveries and female problems involving laparoscopies, D & C's, and hysterectomies. It is not uncommon for a middle-aged woman with fibromyalgia to have had as many as five or six abdominal procedures.

Some researchers have observed high incidence of chronic fatigue and fibromyalgia-like symptoms in women who have had silicone breast implants (Goldman, 1991). Others have reported no association (Sanchez, et al 1995). The best evidence supporting a causal link between silicone and disease is the observation that clinical symptoms stabilize or improve after the removal of implants. Two years after removal, a seventy percent improvement rate is reported (Vasey et al 1994).

The site of injury or trauma is also significant for practitioners working with fibromyalgia and chronic fatigue clients. More data needs to be collected and analyzed in this area, however there are some patterns which may be important for the oriental bodywork therapist or acupuncturist to consider. Cervical and lumbar whiplash injuries, which may or may not involve disk problems; multiple abdominal surgeries; and coccyx injuries seem to be extremely common in fibromyalgia clients.

Some of these injuries may have occurred in childhood and been overlooked or ignored in the treatment of fibromyalgia. When those types of injuries have occurred, and structural imbalances have not been adequately treated, it seems to predispose the body to handle subsequent traumas less efficiently. Thus, old trauma sites which are not producing major symptoms can nonetheless seem to prevent natural self-correction when a new trauma occurs. Thorough intake and assessment should include information about these traumas before beginning oriental bodywork or acupuncture therapy. Releasing abdominal surgical scars and adhesions and balancing spinal and coccyx disharmonies may become important aspects of the treatment.

The spine, the coccyx, and the abdomen are particularly significant for therapists working with the energetic system of Qi and the meridians. The Governing Vessel (Du Mai) and the Bladder meridian (Foot Tai Yang), which are the most Yang pathways in the body, have their trajectories on or alongside the spine, respectively. The Bladder meridian has points (Associated Effects Points, or Back-Shu points) which relate to smooth functioning of the Qi and Organs; the Governing Vessel rules all the Yang energies of the body. When these pathways are disturbed by physical injury there can be a disturbance to the body's energetic field.

The abdomen, especially the lower abdomen, is the source of all the Qi of the body; this energy center is called Dan Tien. If this area is weakened by injury or surgery there is often a profound effect on the body's ability to replenish the Qi. This will be more apparent in individuals who are weak, old, ill, or have repeated surgical events. The abdomen also contains reflex areas for the five major organs: heart, lungs, liver, kidneys and spleen-pancreas-stomach. As with all physiological reflex areas of the body, not only does the area "reflect" the status and health of the related area, but also manipulation or disturbance of a reflex area can influence functioning of the organ.

The coccyx is one of the most important energy centers in the body. Three of the Eight Extra Vessels (Ren Mai, Du Mai, and Chong Mai) meet at the tip of the coccyx (Maciocia, 1989). It lies at the floor of the torso and body cavities. The Bladder meridian and divergents from several of the Yin leg meridians intersect, surround, or travel very near the coccyx. In the Ayurvedic medicine of India, the coccyx is the center of the base chakra. Disturbances to the coccyx may have broad-reaching deleterious effects to the overall health and comfort of the individual. Interestingly, in the author's experience, perhaps as many as fifty percent of fibromyalgia clients have coccyx problems which may be addressed within the scope of oriental bodywork or acupuncture practice.

Emotional trauma

Emotions have long been understood to play a crucial role in health and disease according to oriental views (Teeguarden, 1984; Hammer, 1990). Healthy, balanced emotional expression is desirable, and emotional expression is viewed as another way of discharging build-up of certain kinds of energy in the body. Chronic worry, fear, anger, sadness, and grief are especially damaging to the body's energy and immune systems. Failure to express emotions appropriately can lead to stagnation patterns in which the flow of energy is impaired. Western psychotherapy promotes releasing suppressed emotions and teaching people how to appropriately express feelings.

Many fibromyalgia clients have experienced tragic emotional trauma through the loss of loved ones and the ending of relationships. It is not uncommon for clients to have experienced physical or emotional abuse in the past, or to come from family backgrounds which consistently suppress the free-flowing of emotions. This emotional component may or may not be directly related to depression as part of the presenting clinical picture. Results of a 1991 study, however, did not support a psychopathology model as a primary explanation of the symptoms of primary fibromyalgia syndrome (Ahles, et al, 1991). Thus in most cases, depression is probably secondary rather than primary.

SYMPTOMS OF FIBROMYALGIA AND CHRONIC FATIGUE

These syndromes can produce numerous symptoms. The medical specialty which works with fibromyalgia patients most often (besides primary care physicians) is rheumatology. In 1990, the American College of Rheumatology defined criteria to guide physicians in the diagnosis of fibromyalgia. Those criteria are summarized in Table 1. The tender point locations are shown in Diagram 1.

Different individuals may experience different combinations of symptoms, but there are several cardinal symptoms. These closely correspond to the Center for Disease Control (CDC) diagnostic criteria. Table 2 (at the end of this chapter) lists the symptoms with approximate percentages of diagnosed individuals who have that symptom. In a later chapter, the more important symptoms will be considered from the point of view of Chinese medicine.

Table 1. American College of Rheumatology 1990 Criteria for the Classification of Fibromyalgia

1. <u>History of widespread pain.</u>

Definition: Pain is considered widespread when all the following are present:
- Pain in the left side of the body
- Pain in the right side of the body
- Pain above the waist
- Pain below the waist

In addition, axial skeletal pain (cervical spine or anterior chest or thoracic spine or low back) must be present. In this definition, shoulder and buttock pain is considered as pain for each involved side. "Low back" pain is considered lower segment pain.

2. <u>Pain in 11 of 18 tender point</u> sites on digital palpation.

Definition: Pain, on digital palpation, present in at least 11 of the following 18 sites:

- 1, 2. Occiput: Bilateral, at the suboccipital muscle insertions.
- 3, 4. Low cervical: bilateral, anterior aspects of the intertransverse spaces at C5-C7.
- 5, 6. Trapezius: bilateral, at the midpoint of the upper border.
- 7, 8. Supraspinatus: bilateral, at origins, above scapular spine near the medial border.
- 9, 10. Second rib: bilateral, at the second costochondral junctions, just lateral to the junctions on upper surfaces.
- 11, 12. Lateral epicondyle: bilateral, 2 cm distal to the epicondyles.
- 13, 14. Gluteal: bilateral, in upper outer quadrant of buttocks in anterior fold of muscle.
- 15, 16. Greater trochanter: bilateral, posterior to the trochanteric prominence.
- 17, 18. Knee: bilateral, at the medial fat pad proximal to the joint line.

Digital palpation should be performed with an approximate force of 4 kg. For a tender point to be considered "positive" the subject must state that the palpation was painful. "Tender" is not to be considered "painful."

For classification purposes, patients will be said to have fibromyalgia if both criteria are satisfied. Widespread pain must have been present for at least three months. The presence of a second clinical disorder does not exclude the diagnosis of fibromyalgia.

**Diagram 1. American College of Rheumatology
Fibromyalgia Tender Points**

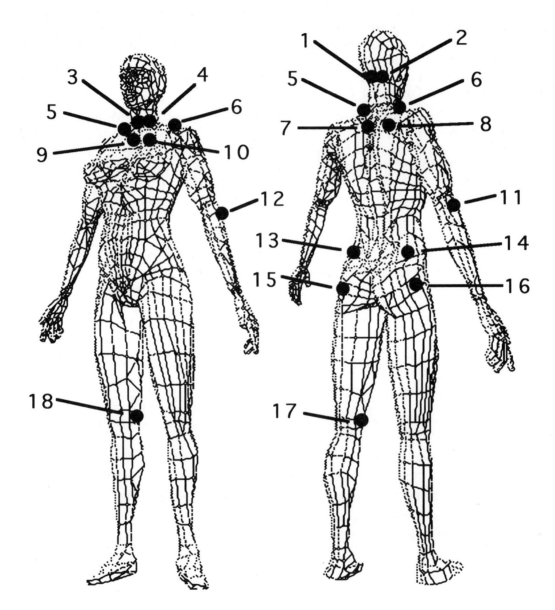

Table 2. Symptoms for Fibromyalgia and Chronic Fatigue Syndrome

	Part 1. CDC Diagnostic Criteria	
	Symptom	% of Clients
1	Fatigue or Exhaustion	95%
2	Headache	90%
3	Post-exertion malaise	80%
4	Short term memory loss	80%
5	Widespread muscle pain	75%
6	Difficulty concentrating	70%
7	Joint pain	65%
8	Lymph node pain	50%
9	Sore throat	50%
	Part 2. Other Common Signs and Symptoms	
10	Non-restorative sleep	90%
11	Fever or sensation of fever	85%
12	Blurry vision	80%
13	Sensitivity to bright lights	80%
14	Light headedness	75%
15	Depression	65%
16	Insomnia	65%
17	Abdominal pain and distension	60%
18	Dry or scratchy eyes	60%
19	Numbness/tingling in extremities	60%
20	Allergies	60%
21	Heart palpitations	55%
22	Night sweats	50%
23	Constipation	40%
24	Flushing rash on face/cheeks	40%
25	Irritable bowel syndrome	40%
26	Muscular weakness	30%
27	Dizziness or vertigo	30%
28	Balance disturbance	30%
29	Panic attacks	30%
30	Eye pain	30%
31	Chills	30%
32	Shortness of breath	30%
33	Bitter or metallic taste in mouth	25%
34	Chemical sensitivities	25%
35	Swollen extremities or eyelids	20%
36	Burning sensation on urination	20%
37	Sexual dysfunction	20%
38	Hair loss	20%
39	Double vision	10%

Chapter 2

Two Paradigms for Health and Healing

Contemporary health care in the United States consists of mainstream allopathic medicine (Western medicine) and a host of alternative or complementary modalities being practised alongside. These approaches are often integrated by individuals seeking help from both mainstream and non-conventional practitioners. In some cases practitioners work together in integrative clinics. Yet it can still be said that there is often marginal acceptance of one by the other. In order to facilitate integrative practice and assist practitioners and clients understand alternative and complementary therapies, it will be helpful to explore the paradigms from which they arise.

ALLOPATHIC (WESTERN MEDICINE) PARADIGM

Western medicine was developed using the scientific method and emphasises that the factors which are important to health must be measurable, usable, predictable, and reproducible. Physical methods such as surgery or substances (drugs, radiation) are used to adjust physiology. Emotions are not regarded as primary in the development of illness. The allopathic (allo= "other", path = "disease") paradigm is based on the belief that the physical world contains the forces that exert the strongest influence upon the body. Illness comes from pathogens, environmental poisons, genetic weaknesses, lack of essential nutrients, accidents, traumas, and breakdown of organ systems as a result of overuse or ageing.

The allopathic paradigm views illness and death as failure; they are problems to be eradicated or postponed into the future. The goal of medical intervention is to eliminate disease and prolong life. The ultimate goal of research is to eliminate disease by eradicating pathogenic organisms, changing genetic weaknesses, or altering physiological processes. Prevention has begun to receive more attention in the latter part of the twentieth century, but education of practitioners and clients has been slow. Prevention currently relies primarily upon vaccination, genetic screening, and other technological approaches rather than stress reduction, diet, or lifestyle modification. Mainstream medicine is starting to recognize how stress and emotional tension disrupt the physiological processes, and therefore contribute to disease, but has not yet embraced this notion that emotional stress and tension form the fundamental matrix within which illness develops. The focus for mainstream medicine is on "cure", which implies eradicating, eliminating, or otherwise ending physical symptoms or disease.

HOLISTIC PARADIGM

The holistic paradigm is the foundation for most alternative and complementary therapies. It is based on the belief that illness results when emotional, physical or spiritual stress becomes overwhelming. The body becomes weakened as a result of prolonged stress, and weakening presents an opportunity for illness to develop. The body reflects or manifests the deeper struggles of the person's entire life. In other words, the energetic aspects of illness precede physical experiences. In this paradigm illness does not happen randomly, but in fact, is usually brewing for months or years prior to the onset of symptoms and medically detectable changes. The characteristics and location of a problem are symbolically important in this paradigm.

Health or disease are the natural outgrowths of how we live life and cope with the demands of our entire life. Most people become involved with holistic approaches (as a client or as a practitioner) through a personal health crisis which generates motivation to seek every level of information about how to work with their health dilemma. A health crisis thus becomes a transformational experience for the person, demanding that he/she evaluate what is and is not working in his/her life, and address the issues. It can also be transformational for family members and friends. This process of inner exploration and change, which often becomes a way of life, ultimately leads the person to a new way of thinking.

In the holistic approach emphasis is on "healing", which is a process that encompasses the person's whole life, not just the medical illness. Symptoms and disease are an outgrowth of the deeper issues. It is possible for healing to occur even in those with "incurable" illnesses, and does not necessarily presuppose the disappearance of the disease. From the holistic view, a person can continue to heal right up to the moment of death, and in fact, death may itself be a healing transformation.

The holistic paradigm is the basis for most, if not all alternative or non-conventional therapies, including traditional Asian medical systems. An underlying principle for holistic approaches is that the causes of illness and disease are ultimately connected to the inner stresses of a person's life. The Taoists call this "Living out of harmony with the natural laws." (See Appendix 3) Emotional, psychological, nutritional and spiritual issues are the central concerns, as they exert the controlling influence on the physical body. In the holistic model matter follows energy.

The term "stress" is a safe bridge term which is both legitimate and non-threatening to most practitioners, and in the broadest sense refers to the human response to life's challenges. The holistic paradigm has existed for millennia and formed the basis for traditional health care systems (native or "folk" medicine, passed down primarily through oral tradition). That it has been emerging and building momentum in the West is indicative of evolutionary change in how people think.

Assumptions of Holistically Based Therapies

1. The body breaks down in response to emotional, psychological and spiritual stresses, as well as physiological stress. Energetic disturbances occur before matter begins to change. This central theme of energetic imbalance is the

1. The body breaks down in response to emotional, psychological and spiritual stresses, as well as physiological stress. Energetic disturbances occur before matter begins to change. This central theme of energetic imbalance is the "unified field theory" of the holistic paradigm in general, and Chinese medicine in particular.

2. In order to heal, unresolved areas of stress need to be uncovered and dealt with effectively. Thus a discovery and learning process must be started. The person must identify the areas of life which are unbalanced, and then he/she must learn how to restore balance within the natural laws.

3. The individual is responsible for his/her own healing process. The practitioner is in the role of facilitator, assistant, educator, partner. Both must have equal status in the healing relationship; there can be no dependency or subordination on the part of the individual. Informed decision making is a crucial part of this dynamic.

4. Therapies assist the person in understanding their stress and tension patterns, and then assist in releasing these patterns. Oriental acutherapy and other touch therapies are especially valuable for the process of increasing body awareness.

5. Success of therapy rests upon two key points:
   a. The individual's courage and commitment to honestly evaluate
   his life. Self -examination is the catalyst for change (Table 3).

   b. The person's ability to make choices that authentically
   empower the self and give access to his inner resources.

Table 3. Self Examination Leads to Personal Change

Self ========>	Reveals what is ======>	Problems ======>	Attention ======>	Choice
Examination	not working in one's life	demand attention	activates choice	brings change

Maximum effects require awareness on the part of the client. The person must be re-educated to use thoughts, emotions, and images to change the body. The energetic model postulates that Qi follows thought. Learning to command the mind to direct thoughts and images is an important step.

6. The holistic paradigm acknowledges the concept of thought-form. This is the notion that thoughts are "things" and possess energy which activates them and directs them to manifest into the physical world. They energize us to do one thing or another, and direct physiological activity. Their power is released through "belief", and not just mental understanding. Thought-forms are shared systems of consciousness which can be tapped into and operate as the "realities" which govern our lives, for better or worse. A paradigm consists of a set of thought-forms which are shared by practitioners and clients and accepted as truth. The paradigm becomes real, effective and dynamic in a person's life in proportion to his/her acceptance of the thought-forms as truth. Examples of key thought-forms in holistic health approaches:

- We create our own reality
- We co-create reality with those we interact with
- Energy follows thought
- Illness has potential for positive personal transformation and can be a catalyst for spiritual growth
- Healing is a higher process than curing because it invokes greater awareness on the part of the client

7. Besides any therapeutic interventions the client may be receiving, there are additional factors which influence the process of healing:

- The individual's motivation to begin self-examination
- The individual's ability to engage in mental/emotional skills with clarity and focus
- The individual's aptitude for inner work
- Intensity, duration and type of illness
- Nature of the underlying stresses connected to the illness condition
- Competence, experience, and wisdom of therapists/instructors
- What's going on "the rest of the time" when the person is not in a therapy session- fears, anger, negative belief patterns, destructive behaviors

Robert Dilts (1990) proposed a simple model to assist practitioners and clients in understanding the dynamics of change, including physical healing (Table 4). The model is simple and straightforward and captures the essential ingredients needed for change and healing.

Table 4. Dilts Model for Change

```
                 Want To
                 /   \
                /     \
        How To---Chance To
```

First the individual needs to have motivation to change; he or she must "want to". At the most basic level motivation causes the individual to seek help or not. Fears and doubts may also interfere with the person's ability or willingness to take action. Input from significant others, secondary gain and beliefs about the possibility for change or healing all influence the "want to" part of the process. (See Chapter 9 for more on secondary gain) If activity and movement are blocked at this stage, the person may never get any further in the process of change or healing.

The second phase is the "how to" stage. This stage encompasses such things as deciding what therapeutic modalities to use, which therapist or physician to go to, and the development of skills for lifestyle modification and other personal changes. For example, someone might recognize the benefit of whole food diet, and have interest and motivation to change his diet, but may not know how to go about it. At this stage, education is the key factor which enables the individual to make use of his motivation. In many situations a person may know how to do something, and believe that it would be beneficial, but lack the motivation to pursue it. Exercise programs are a good example of this. "Want to" and "How To" must both be considered in order to enable the client to start a change process.

The third phase is the "chance to" phase. In the beginning, one's skills may be rather poor as they start the learning process. Mistakes, relapses and errors are an inherent part of learning a new skill or behavior. Whether the person has decided to work with diet, exercise, meditation, self-acutherapy or massage, there will be a learning curve as they begin to incorporate the new skill into their life.

Another aspect of the "chance to" phase is to allow enough time for the therapeutic process to work. Sometimes people are discouraged when, after three of four sessions of acutherapy or after exercising for one month, they have not accrued massive changes. They may recognize that some symptoms are less and they feel somewhat better overall, but are not where they expected to be. Education is a key factor here. Practitioners must help the client understand how the process of healing unfolds. Many times there are indications of healing which a client may not recognize as such. "Healing Crisis's" are an example in which the person may actually feel worse for awhile, or old symptoms may temporarily resurface. It is a sad loss when an individual who has the motivation and the know-how discontinues his good work because he loses patience with the process, or does not know how to read the signs of progress along the way.

8. There are four general categories of imbalances which can lead to symptoms and disease. These are interconnected and influence one another and each responds better to different kinds of therapies. It is beneficial for the therapist to identify which are the key factors in the client's health problems.

- Structural/mechanical problems
- Emotional/spiritual problems
- Nutritional/systemic problems
- Electromagnetic/environmental problems

9. Core problems and obstacles to healing must be identified and addressed. Among the more common ones:

a. Lack of courage to evaluate what is working or not working in one's life. Self-exploration can be a terrifying process, because it forces us to redefine the very "reality" we hold as truth. To break down one's belief system and then rebuild it according to higher truths is a spiritual process which many resist. We seem to instinctively know that undergoing this process will disrupt and unravel the very fabric of our lives, potentially leading to emotional upheaval and changes in relationships and values.

   b.   Denial of effect of stressors on health and well-being. Few people want to give up their comfortable and familiar habits. Denial surrounding addictive behaviors is legendary. Smokers, alcoholics and other addicts usually have to confront their denial of their addiction as a first step to recovery. No less extreme are the attachments people have to soda pop, meat, sugar and other unhealthy foods. Denial of other types of stressors such as relationships and jobs are also difficult to face in the beginning, and people often maintain denial about their dysfunctional relationships. Battered wives who return to their violent husbands are an example of this type of denial.

   c. Lack of skills for introspection or self-examination. Self-examination requires ability to discern among various choices, to receive internal and external feedback, to have adequate communication skills, to be able to access and utilize resources to facilitate change and healing.

   d. Undeveloped will power. Implementing new lifestyle choices such as diet, exercise, meditation, training for a new career, or giving up addictions require personal will power. Many have experienced the difficulty of maintaining a commitment to a new regime, or have relapsed from addictions to cigarettes, sugar, caffeine, alcohol and other drugs. It also takes will power to commit to maintaining appropriate personal boundaries, for example when one tends to be a rescuer or a victim. These habitual patterns can only change through perseverance, observation of self and through receiving feedback. Handling changes for a healthy lifestyle are much smoother when one has developed self-control and will power.

   The phrase "Dark Night of the Soul" was coined by St. John of the Cross to describe the feelings of isolation, abandonment, helplessness and surrender encountered when one starts to move from a spiritually unawakened state to an awakened one. This metaphor applies to any one who embarks upon a spiritual path; healing can be an example. Entering the "dark night" requires will power and faith. Not every person is ready or able to accept what the holistic field has to offer. The acceptance of personal empowerment is a big responsibility and can be frightening to people who have lived their whole lives with others making their decisions for them. Many individuals and "the system" still operate on a distribution of power which causes the client to be in the position of subordination to outside forces and influences.

Diagram 2. Dark Night of the Soul

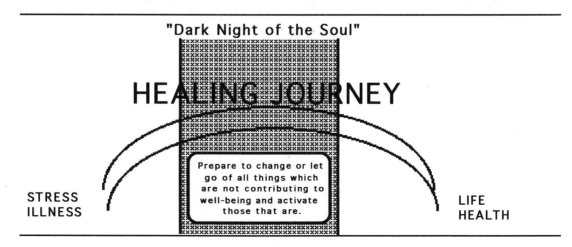

"Dark Night of the Soul"

HEALING JOURNEY

Prepare to change or let go of all things which are not contributing to well-being and activate those that are.

STRESS
ILLNESS

LIFE
HEALTH

10. Changes in perceptions frequently occur as a result of healing work. When people begin to encounter their own wholeness they begin to experience a profound transformation in their perspective on their lives. The changes in perception then further facilitate the process. The individual gradually finds that his life has changed in meaningful ways as his perceptions shift. Some of the perceptions which change can include:

Out of control	------------>	Being in control
Beyond help/hope	------------>	Sense of possibility
Fear, anger	------------>	Acceptance, forgiveness
World as dangerous	------------>	Sense of inner peace

11. Illness often functions as a messenger in ones' life.

a. Discovery of an illness can start a transformational process. For some individuals it may be the starting point of a journey which leads to that person's spiritual purpose in life. Many who have become practitioners and teachers in holistic therapies, including oriental medicine, learned that their own health challenges and the process of inner exploration were a starting point which ultimately led them to study and become a practitioner.

b. Illness or disability present challenges to act in ways that promote health. This involves shedding of illusions about former behaviors, making purposeful decisions, and developing will power. Thus, illness becomes a teacher for living in closer harmony with the natural laws.

c. Illness, disability or injury frequently directs one to redefine one's identity. What a person accepted as true about himself must often shift. Most people experience a version of this when the effects of ageing begin to develop in middle age. The changes can be very sudden, as with disabling injury, or can develop gradually over months or years. In either case, illness teaches us about ourselves.

d. Illness often causes the individual to re-prioritize personal values. Things which once seemed important often diminish when one is facing a chronic or potentially life-threatening illness. In this way, illness can help a person awaken to deeper realities. What's new for most Western people is the awareness that our thoughts create our reality. The truth of that notion has been active for thousands of years, has been recognized by other cultures, and forms the basis for all traditional medical systems.

A Vision for Health Care in the Twenty-First Century

- Health care practitioners will be knowledgeable about both allopathic and holistic ways of approaching health challenges.

- Health care practitioners will work integratively, utilizing all the approaches which may be beneficial for a client. Several types of therapy will be offered in each clinic, including mainstream and holistic methods.

- Less emphasis on "heroic" medical treatments and more emphasis on wellness and prevention.

- Higher standards of training and licensing for therapists in massage therapy, homeopathy, herbal medicine, aromatherapy, hypnotherapy and others.

- Individuals (clients and practitioners) will be activating healthy lifestyle principles and stress management strategies into every-day living. These include whole foods nutrition, exercise, meditation, and other naturalistic interventions before using drugs or surgery.

- Pharmaceutical companies will shift emphasis to growing plants for herbal and essential oil production. Responsible disclosure of all benefits and hazards of products will be standard procedure.

- Individuals will become fully informed about their choices for working with a health challenge, and be empowered to take charge of their health strategies. Practitioners are team-mates, facilitators, and educators.

- Medical insurance will become less important as people learn to care for themselves, remain healthier longer, and utilize naturalistic interventions which are much less costly. Clients will come to value their health so they are willing to pay for beneficial therapies out-of-pocket. Medical insurance companies may adopt strategies of life insurance, providing investment return to insureds when health benefits are not used.

- Health care becomes less a political/ economic issue, and more a humanistic, personalized, individual issue.

Chapter 3

Personal Characteristics and Health

A cornerstone of the holistic paradigm is the connection among all levels of functioning: mind, body, emotions and spirit. Several of the Chinese medical models have robust descriptions of the mental, emotional and spiritual aspects of human functioning: Five Elements, Six Divisions and the Five "Shen" are examples. In the West, models for understanding mental and emotional processes fall mostly in the domain of psychology and sociology. Mainstream Western medicine has only begun to take interest in these matters since approximately 1980 when the connection between "Type A" personality and heart attack became widely known.

Numerous models have been developed and reported in the psychological literature since the late 1960's. Many of these propose links between mental or emotional processes, stress, and health outcomes. Some have focused on specialized areas such as heart disease or cancer. Others have more generalized applications and can be helpful for the practitioner working with chronic disharmonies such as fibromyalgia and chronic fatigue. This chapter includes several different models which have been to understand chronic illnesses.

The practitioner who is familiar with these models can frequently observe patterns of stress, behavior or thinking that may block progress in a client who is doing "everything right". Frequently a practitioner may have a client who has put great effort into lifestyle changes such as diet, exercise, sunlight and supplements, and yet progress is still very slow. This is the time to consider some of the models from this chapter, and help the client identify and work with some of the types of stress and internal patterns that may be preventing improvement. Working with the tension patterns of the body through acupuncture, acupressure, or massage while simultaneously helping the client understand her own tension patterns of thought and emotion can release the barriers to healing and profoundly support the person's personal development.

Attributional Styles

Dr. Martin Seligman, (Seligman et al 1979; Peterson et al 1982) described two approaches to life, which he called "attributional styles". He found these correlate highly with health and recovery from illness in a study with cancer patients. He called the two types Pessimistic and Optimistic. Characteristics of each are summarized in Table 5.

Table 5. Attributional Styles

The Pessimist	The Optimist
Self-blame in negative events	No self-blame for negative events
Belief that effects of negative events will last a long time	Belief that effects of negative events are limited in time
Belief that effects of a negative event will influence many or all areas of life	Belief that effects of negative events have limited influence on life areas
Catastrophizing	More balanced perspective
Hopelessness, depression, self-preoccupation	Problem solving; identifying and employing useful resources
More likely to manifest symptoms when faced with negative events	Less likely to manifest symptoms when faced with negative events
Hormonal/immune changes characteristic of disease susceptibility	Less changes in hormonal/ immune system functioning under stress
In a study of cancer patients, the more pessimistic patients died earlier	In a study of cancer patients, the more optimistic patients lived longer

It is usually easy to determine if a client has an optimistic or pessimistic style by listening to what they say during the intake and in conversation during therapy sessions. Also the practitioner can ask simple questions to gather information, listening not to the particular details of the response, but to the tendency to either of these styles. Example questions could include:

* Tell me about your experiences with other practitioners.
* What do you believe is the deepest underlying cause of your problems?
* What type of outcome do you expect in regard to your health?
* How do things generally turn out for you in other areas of life?
* What are some of the things you can do for yourself to improve your health?

Self-Efficacy

Dr. Albert Bandura of Stanford University Medical School defined "self-efficacy" as the belief in one's own ability to exercise control over specific events in one's life, and confidence in one's own ability to influence outcomes even when new, unpredictable, stressful events occur (Bandura 1977). Higher degrees of self-efficacy have been shown to be a predictor of positive health outcomes for many health challenges, including heart attack, arthritis, and in making changes such as quitting smoking. Table 6 gives examples of kinds of thoughts which are characteristic of people with high and low self-efficacy.

Table 6. Examples of Low and High Self-Efficacy

Low Self Efficacy Thinking	High Self Efficacy Thinking
"I can't help it"	"I am responsible"
"I don't know what to do"	"I'll find a way"
"Who can do it for me?"	"I can do this"
"Show me what to do"	"I'll figure it out"
"You do it first"	"Let me try"
"I don't know what caused it"	"I think I see my role in creating this"
"I wonder how I can avoid this"	"I wonder what I will learn from this"
"The situation is hopeless"	"The situation is a challenge"
"There's nothing I can do"	"I have resources I can draw from"
"I am a helpless victim"	"I am in charge of my life"
"What do you think I should do?"	"I'll think it over and decide what to do"

Many clients who seek assistance from health care practitioners are looking for someone who can "fix" their problems or "cure" their illness. They behave as if the causes and solutions to their problems are external, and improvement comes to them through a practitioner "giving them something" for the problem, or doing something to them. These are people with low "self-efficacy", and both mainstream and non-conventional health care practitioners see such individuals. They frequently have been to numerous practitioners and specialists seeking a "magic bullet" for their ailments. They are often discouraged and disillusioned because they can't seem to find the one remedy or doctor who can solve their problems. Working with these individuals can be quite challenging, and the task is to help the person come to believe in his/her own ability to change the situation. Quite often they are helpless and dependent in other areas of their lives also.

Appropriate homework can be an excellent way to begin helping the person develop higher self-efficacy. Reading assignments, stretches or exercises, or taking herbs or supplements may be good places to start. Encourage the person to evaluate his/her experience and start to do trouble-shooting. Frequently stating that "No one know your body as well as you do", and "No one knows what you need as well as you do." and other positive affirmations can plant suggestions that will empower the person to develop higher self-efficacy.

Stress Hardiness

•Dr. Suzanne Kobasa and colleagues researched the connection of personality traits, stress, and illness. (Kobasa, 1979, 1982, 1983) She defined a characteristic called "Stress-Hardiness". Stress-Hardy individuals consistently displayed three characteristics:

- •<u>Control:</u> Being in control (at cause) in one's own life.
- •<u>Commitment:</u> Being fully engaged in the healing process, giving full effort, devotion to meaningful work and family.
- •<u>Challenge:</u> Seeing change as a natural part of life; opportunity for learning and growth.

Since chronic illness is, in itself, a powerful stressor for most people, developing better stress-hardiness can be a valuable strategy. Living with chronic fatigue and/or chronic discomfort can easily erode the stress-hardiness an individual may have had prior to becoming ill. Certain stress patterns also can contribute to the perpetuation and exacerbation of symptoms. Stress and symptoms are frequently part of an escalating spiral; stress makes symptoms worse, and worsening symptoms increase stress. The following list summarizes common stress patterns. The practitioner can explore these ideas with the client, helping her identify patterns which affect her. Then she can work to find solutions and positive changes to relieve stress and restore stress-hardiness.

SIGNIFICANT STRESS PATTERNS
WHICH CONTRIBUTE TO ILLNESS

1. Unresolved or deeply consuming emotional, psychological, or spiritual stress. This need not be the result of a dramatic event, nor is the event necessarily observable by others. The trigger could be a one-time event or it can be an ongoing or long term influence. An unresolved event can be very old (childhood origin) or more recent.

2. Negative belief patterns which dominate or control one's reality. These can be beliefs about life, people, the self, luck, God, career, or just about anything else. Empowering belief patterns promote good health.

3. Taking life too seriously, including lack of humor and fun. Seeing the humorous side of things and laughing frequently make the stressful events of life less powerful to induce negative changes. Equanimity, the view that events are not inherently good nor bad, but simply opportunities which provide the lessons of life, is a trait of people who are highly developed spiritually and personally.

4. Inability to give and/or receive love. Human love and warmth are necessary ingredients for a rich and healthy life.

5. Lack of power and choice in one's life. Giving up our free will to "powerful others", which may be individuals or institutions, dis-empowers the individual and forms the medium in which anger, rage, resentment, and low self-esteem can develop. Having personal power and

choice include openness to compromise, altering our plans, and being flexible and responsive to the needs of others.

6.   Failure to attend to needs of the physical body, including exercise, high-quality food and water, sufficient rest, healthy touch, and breaking free of substance abuse.

7.   Suffering which accompanies absence of meaning or purpose in one's life. Depression, despair, loneliness, and feelings of worthlessness result.

8.   Tendency toward denial. The failure to recognize and acknowledge what isn't working in one's life is a sure way to become ill. We are meant to learn and grow through life's challenges, and denial blocks energy and keeps us stuck. Change cannon begin until we first have awareness of the problems, both internally and externally.

LIFE CHALLENGES FOR OPTIMIZING PERSONAL HEALTH

Life presents numerous challenges to every person. Most, if not all spiritual traditions regard life's challenges as the reason for living and as the true teachers that usher us along our spiritual paths. Four of the major life challenges that will be encountered by most people are considered in this section. Each of these four has a connection to health because they determine how one may attempt to resolve a health challenge, how they may live with chronic symptoms, and how they may facilitate others who are dealing with health concerns.

Power (Self empowerment)

The development of personal power is a universal theme in every person's life, and follows a predictable pattern.

Symbolic Power

First we learn to associate power with external symbols such as money, possessions, social status, control of others, approval and attention from others, titles, awards, and degrees. Focus on external objects is indicative of what is lacking internally; this is the "mirror effect".

Examples of symbolic power:

• Using money for power relates to one's self-value system

• Using objects for power relates to lack of well-formed self-identity

• Personal dominance used for power reveals one's inner inferiority

• Titles, awards, and degrees are used to elevate one's self esteem and prove value or worth to others through accomplishments and achievements

- Social or political status used for power show ignorance or inattention to the concept of unity and interconnection of all people

The stronger one's obsession with power symbols, the greater lack of authentic power. Other indicators of weak personal power include criticism, gossip, devaluing other's opinions, need to be right, confrontational attitude or domineering in work or personal relationships. Physical symptoms which reflect chronic attachment to external power symbols or seeking self-empowerment through external gratification include ulcers, hypertension, and migraines. Those who habitually have their personal power negated or diminished through the actions of others, who find the world threatening, who frequently feel intimidated, or who are being used or taken advantage of by "powerful others" are more prone to developing cancer (Temoshok,199?.)

Authentic Power

As one develops a deep regard for his/her own self esteem, personal dignity, living in harmony with others and with nature, self-love, and love of all living things, he/she approaches the level of authentic power. Then there is no need to dominate or control others; money and material objects become tools for improving living conditions, education, healing for all; and genuine leadership emerges. Unfortunately, although serious illness, financial ruin, ending of relationships, and other life crises can often be the catalyst for a person to start to develop authentic power, many people never attain authentic power in their lives. Attributional style and self-efficacy, discussed earlier in this chapter, both bear relationship to how one meets the challenge of self-empowerment.

Responsibility

The second major challenge is developing a willingness to take responsibility for oneself, including quality of life, attitudes, failures and successes, and for one's own health. As a person develops responsibility there is no longer need for blaming other people or circumstances for what is happening in one's life. Releasing self-blame and learning an attitude of forgiveness are aspects of developing responsibility. When a person makes a commitment to assume total responsibility for everything that has happened or will happen to him/her, he/she also must be willing to develop the courage and honesty to make decisions and take actions which will lead to the desired outcomes. Being responsible means there are no more excuses, blaming or "guilt trips", and the person moves to a position of authority in his/her own life. This step necessitates the release of victim thinking and moves the person into the causal position in cause-and-effect relationships. Before learning responsibility, the individual is at the EFFECT of external causes:

Cause =======> EFFECT

After learning responsibility, individual is the CAUSE of events in his life:

CAUSE =======> Effect

Each of these life challenges has a "shadow side", and some people get into trouble with responsibility by nominating themselves to "be responsible" for other people's quality of life, attitudes, decisions and so on. Being overly responsible can lead to issues of control and domination, and can deny another person the opportunity to develop his own personal power and responsibility. The development of responsibility is often triggered by an event involving disillusionment or betrayal by people or institutions one has depended upon to make decisions and govern one's life.

Wisdom

Wisdom is the willingness and awareness to learn from all situations of life. This type of experiential learning leads to the development of a "larger picture" of life, and is a key to breaking the cycles of repeated mistakes or decisions in life. Developing wisdom requires the person to learn to "step outside" of him/her self to observe the overall dynamics of the situation. A wise question to ask in every situation, especially unpleasant or uncomfortable ones, is "What is this experience teaching me?" Developing wisdom is another component in releasing victim consciousness, bitterness, anger, frustration, and fears. Failure to learn the lesson of wisdom keeps one's life from moving forward, keeps one stuck in increasingly more dramatic examples of the lesson that's being missed, and is the root of many disharmonies and illnesses. Health problems can be exceedingly powerful teachers of wisdom.

Love

Disharmonies involving inability to learn the lessons of love include adopting substitutes for love, such as material or manipulating others with "love" ("I'm doing this for your own good"; "I'm doing this because I love you"; "if I didn't love you I wouldn't...."). Loneliness, resentment over rejection, fear of being loved, fear of NOT being loved, repeated disappointments in personal relationships, and guilt over not fulfilling the expectations of others are all patterns one can fall into while learning the lessons of love. Heartbreak, hurt feelings, loneliness, feelings of not belonging and detachment are all indications that this lesson is still in progress.

Health challenges can be a great teacher for the lesson of love. Illness or injury frequently alters one's self-image, and therefore one's ability for self-love. Working with or living with others who have disabilities or health challenges can be another version of the lesson. For practitioners, being able to accept clients and work with them unconditionally, even when they have self-destructive behaviors, weak personal power, low responsibility, and poorly developed wisdom can be an opportunity to develop power, responsibility, wisdom, and love in ourselves.

PERSONALITY AND THE IMPERSONAL SELF

The "personality" starts its development in infancy. It is a way to meet survival needs, and a way to enter into relationships with care-givers, siblings, and later one's peer group and society in general. It reflects early childhood "programming" from the family and culture that raises an individual; this is one's "tribal belief system". Tribal belief systems could be thought of as "relative truths" in that they are agreed upon and acted upon as if they were true within that group. For the members of that social system, they give the boundaries of what is real and unreal, possible and impossible, permissible and not permissible.

The personality, as it develops within cultural and familial guidelines, is the source of what is called "EGO PAIN", which comes from the struggle to maintain the system of illusions learned from the "tribe". Among the illusions one comes to accept as true are self-worth, his role and roles of others in the family, how relationships work, religious beliefs, and what to expect our life, among many others.

A person who begins a path of personal evolution beyond the beliefs and customs taught by his "tribe" will inevitably experience a heavy dose of ego pain as he/she recognizes the disillusionment that accompanies the failure of what he once believed to be true. It is, in fact, often the failure of expectations which launches the individual into a search for higher truths. When the tribal belief system fails it can leave the individual feeling isolated, detached, and confused. The person has, for the first time, encountered the "Dark Night of the Soul" (See Chapter 2).

"Toto, I don't think we're in Kansas anymore."

As a person starts her/his journey to the discovery of greater "truths" the experience of "SOUL PAIN" starts to manifest. This occurs as acceptance, surrender or release occur, as he begins to learn the truth about himself. He begins to let go of the childhood persona and discover his "Impersonal Self":

"Guess what, Mom and Dad; I have realized I am NOTHING like you!
"Somehow I just don't seem to fit in any more."
"This isn't how I thought it would be."

He starts to awaken to deeper realities and the shedding of illusions and discover that there is a higher purpose in life.

"I need some time to think and "find myself".
"There's got to be more to life than THIS"
"I want something more than just a job"

Health is one result of a commitment to live a more conscious, responsible, and empowered life, through the development of the impersonal self. That is the challenge which overwhelms many people who could change their lives, and they even know some of the things they need to do.

"It's alot of work."

This process of changing awareness is the beginning of transformation of the personality to the impersonal self, or spiritual self. Characteristics of each are shown in Table 7.

One of the expectations which is frequently shattered is the illusion that we have a right to perfect health and eternal youth. The person who encounters chronic illness such as chronic fatigue or fibromyalgia is often faced with a struggle to move away from the narrow belief system of the tribe, and toward a belief system which includes a broader view of health and its ramifications. This can be a catalyst for starting to develop the impersonal self, and often such an experience leads to major life changes.

Table 7. Personality and Impersonal Self

Personality	Impersonal Self
Ego-centered view of the world	Connected to all humanity and life
Self as center of the world	Self as part of a larger world
Fears, needs, insecurities	Higher purpose and reasoning
Attachment to externals	Equanimity and transcendence
Life as struggle	Life as teacher
Will to live	Will to heal

EXERCISE: HEALTHY AND UNHEALTHY PATTERNS

The two lists that follow summarize many of the concepts presented in this chapter. Individuals with chronic fatigue or fibromyalgia and practitioners who work with them are encouraged to do an honest self evaluation from these two lists. An excellent way to work with them is to write a paragraph or two about each item. Recall examples from your life relating to the items, ideas for change, what others have said in regard to a particular item, and other thoughts. This may be done over a period of time, working with only one or two of the items each day. Then consider changes you may want to change in the interest of better health.

Unhealthy Patterns:

_____ I have thoughts or beliefs that support helpless/hopeless feelings
_____ I feel as if I have lost control in my own life
_____ I frequently feel or express hostility and cynicism
_____ I feel a lack of enthusiasm or commitment for life's challenges
_____ I am frequently unable to express feelings
_____ Anger/ Irritability/ Fears are dominant themes in my life
_____ I tend to be overly serious and self-obsessed
_____ I feel isolation and detachment from others
_____ I focus on the past and future with guilt, worry, and see problems
_____ I tend to hold on to negatives for an overly long time
_____ I easily allow negatives to generalize to many contexts in my life
_____ I think of life as threatening, terrorizing, dangerous
_____ I feel lack of purpose; life seems meaningless

Health-Promoting Patterns:

_____ I have many empowering beliefs
_____ I can easily let go of negative events, people, circumstances
_____ I am at choice; I am the primary causal agent in one's own life
_____ I have a good sense of humor, being able to laugh at myself
_____ I have commitment, motivation, interest in life's challenges
_____ I see obstacles and problems as challenges
_____ For me, life is a positive adventure, a journey of learning
_____ I feel a strong sense of connection and support with others
_____ Life has purpose and is richly meaningful to me
_____ I am increasingly developing the ability to forgive and let go
_____ In most circumstances, I am able to choose peace rather than chaos
_____ I can forgive others for past wounds and let go of pain from my history

Chapter 4

Introduction to Chinese Medicine and Acutherapy

This chapter introduces acutherapy (acupuncture and oriental bodywork therapy) as viable methods for helping clients with fibromyalgia and chronic fatigue. Chinese medicine provides a different description of human functioning, and therefore, different therapeutic tools for dealing with health challenges. Acutherapy is the stimulation of the energetic points (acupoints) and meridians on the surface of the body to produce changes in the amount or distribution of the Qi, or vital energy which determines health or illness. The points and meridians can be stimulated by pressing (acupressure), needling (acupuncture), heat (moxibustion), magnets (magnet acutherapy), and other methods. Several of these methods are discussed in greater detail in Chapter 6.

Chinese medicine is based on the principle of dynamic equilibrium, or balance, between those phenomena which are classified as Yang and the phenomena which are classified as Yin. Yang phenomena include Qi, (the vital energy), and Shen (the spirit, or consciousness). Yang energy is hotter, dryer, more active, more non-physical and more expansive than Yin energy. Yin phenomena include Blood, body fluids, and Essence, or the physical makeup of the body. Yin energy is cooler, moister, less active, more physical, and more contractive than Yang energy.

According to Chinese medical theory, robust and vital health leading to long, productive, happy lifetime results from abundance of the Vital Substances called Qi (Yang) and Blood (Yin) flowing evenly and steadily in the organs, tissues, and energetic channels, or meridians, of the body. Yin and Yang must be balanced with one another. Illness develops when there is imbalance in these vital substances, including insufficient amounts, inadequate blocked flow, or incorrect direction of flow of the vital substances throughout the body.

"Organs" have a different meaning in Chinese medicine than for Western medicine. Even though the same names (heart, liver, lungs, etc.) are used the Chinese meanings for these terms are much broader than in Western medicine. For Chinese medicine the name of an organ includes not only the anatomical structure, but also the meridian and the energetic functions attributed to that organ. Organs have their presence throughout the body, not just in one location in the body. To make this distinction the organ names will be capitalized when referring to the Chinese concept, and in lower case for the Western anatomical definition of the organ. The Liver, for example, includes the anatomical liver organ, the Liver meridian, and functions such as "storing the Blood," "insuring the smooth spreading of Qi throughout the body", and "opening into the eyes".

"Task of practitioner"

The task of the practitioner of oriental modalities, is to ascertain the nature of the deficiency or blockage, and then assist the body in achieving better balance of Yin and Yang by building strength and clearing blockages. Assessment techniques such as pulse and tongue diagnosis, palpation of specific areas on the body, visibly observable characteristics such as skin color or posture, and information given verbally by the client help the practitioner identify the imbalance that is causing the symptoms and complaints of the client. The results of the assessment assist the practitioner in determining where and how the Qi and Blood are unbalanced.

Treatments

Treatments consist of manipulating the Qi and Blood through the acupoints along the energy pathways. Manipulation can be done in a variety of ways including acupuncture needles, massage, finger pressure, movement therapy such as stretching and range-of-motion, heat, magnets, ion pellets and electro-acupuncture (Deluze et al, 1992). The Qi and Blood can also be influenced by the use of specifically prescribed Chinese herbal formulations as well. Whether therapy is by herbs or physical manipulation of the Qi or both, assessment must be thorough to arrive at the best therapeutic strategy for any individual.

by Chinese formulas

Chinese Medicine is a holistic approach and primarily strives to treat the root cause of the problem, whether it manifests as physical symptoms, emotional symptoms, or both. It is understood that either physical or emotional upsets can lead to imbalances which we call illness or symptoms. Symptoms are seen as clues to help the practitioner identify the underlying problem. Treating symptoms, while often regarded as secondary in the long-term treatment plan, is usually worked into early treatments in order to give the client relief from bothersome or painful symptoms and to release energy which may be used to balance the underlying condition. As treatment progresses, diminishing or changing symptoms guide the practitioner and serve as feedback and confirmation for both practitioner and client that the treatments are effective.

Chinese medicine treats root cause of problem

As the healing process occurs over time the underlying disharmony can shift in both nature and severity. The practitioner is always re-assessing and changing the details of the treatment with each session. As the disharmony changes the treatment points or techniques will be modified also. Different layers of the imbalance can unfold and present themselves like layers seen when peeling an onion.

Chinese medicine recognizes that the same symptom or group of symptoms can arise from a variety of different underlying disharmonies. This means that person with a symptom presentation that is diagnosed as "fibromyalgia syndrome" by Western medicine may have a very unique and different disharmony from other individuals, just as his or her personal history and genetic constitution are different from every other. There are, however, some general tendencies that can guide the client and practitioner using oriental therapies to treat fibromyalgia syndrome.

INTERPRETATION OF SYMPTOMS BY TRADITIONAL CHINESE MEDICINE

A discussion of the cardinal signs and symptoms of fibromyalgia syndrome here will point toward major Yin/Yang and Blood/Qi disharmonies as defined by traditional Chinese medicine. In addition to the cardinal signs and symptoms, there are a number of other common correlated complaints which many, but not necessarily all, patients may have as part of their presenting pattern (Waylonis and Heck, 1992; Hudson, et al 1992).

Cardinal Signs and Symptoms

1. _Widespread body pain which effects muscles more than joints_

This is present continually or intermittently in all fibromyalgia clients, and is the cardinal symptom for fibromyalgia. Some people report that discomfort varies in intensity, quality, and location, or is vague and migrating, or is deep, nagging and aching. Others experience discomfort in fixed locations. Muscle cramps are common. The pain seems to be present both during movement and inactivity. For most people, some days are worse than others.

Severity of muscular pain is frequently correlated with several variables: 1) emotional or physical stress, 2) lack of sufficient rest, 3) lack of appropriate exercise 4) aggravating activities (Waylonis, 1994), 5) lack of purposeful stretching, and 6) low pressure weather patterns and storm conditions, or cold and damp weather. Many clients report the sensation of muscle tightness or cramping. It is common for there to be abnormal texture, tightness, ropiness, or lack of resiliency to the muscle tissue at the sites of the classical tender points and throughout the painful areas.   There is often a quality of lumpiness and nodules in the painful areas. In most cases range-of-motion is somewhat limited, and the client will complain of feeling stiff or tight during joint mobilization.

Widespread body pain is common in the general population; one study in England found the prevalence of chronic widespread pain was 11.2% in a group of over 2000 subjects (Croft et al., 1993.)   The oriental bodywork therapist or acupuncturist is apt to see many clients who present with such pain but have not been medically diagnosed with fibromyalgia syndrome; fibromyalgia should be suspected in these cases.

Morning stiffness is a common complaint and is related to the musculoskeletal discomfort described. Long periods without movement contribute to pain, whether this occurs during the night-time sleep period, or even while awake during the day. The Chinese system classifies morning as the time when Yang energy is rising, so if a person has a pattern of Qi stagnation, they may feel their symptoms more strongly during this time of day. After they arise and move about, the stiffness decreases as the Qi moves more smoothly.

For the practitioner of Chinese medicine, this description of pain points to a blockage in the flows of Qi or Blood in the body, Blockages can result from stagnation of Qi or Blood, or from the presence of a pernicious influence (Damp, Wind, Cold or Heat for example) obstructing the energetic meridians. Dull aching, non-specific pain is characteristic of deficiency type stagnation, and sharp, stabbing, fixed pain such as appendicitis or angina indicate an excess blocking the meridians. In fibromyalgia, Dampness is the most common pernicious influence.

2. *Chronic fatigue.*

Fatigue and pain are frequently inseparable in clients presenting with fibromyalgia syndrome. Pain in and of itself is very energy-draining, and fatigue leads to reduction of activity for most people, therefore a cyclical pattern develops. Acupuncture and bodywork are effective in breaking the pain-fatigue cycle so that clients may be able to resume appropriate stretching and/or gentle exercise such as walking, swimming, Yoga, or Tai Chi therapeutic exercise. Regular use of these or similar activities should be a part of the client's ongoing self-management regime.

Fatigue is a sign of depletion of Qi in the body. Much of the benefit of acutherapy comes from tonification of Qi in general, and specific Organ Qi if the practitioner is able to make diagnostic distinctions at that level. One of the advantages of shiatsu, tuina and other hands-on modalities is that whole-body treatments can be given, thus making it less critical to arrive at an exact assessment. The acupuncturist will be selecting a few treatment points to use so identification of specific imbalances is much more important.

3. *Sleep Disturbances.*

Sleep disturbances can include several energy-draining patterns, including insomnia (inability to fall asleep, or waking often during the night, or waking very early in the morning with inability to go back to sleep), dream-disturbed sleep, or non-restorative sleep. Some clients report that their pain keeps them awake, or causes them to awaken during the night, and disturbance in the sleep cycle probably contributes to their syndrome because of lack of restful sleep. Sleep deprivation also contributes to the emotional and psychological stress that can easily increase when sleep is not restorative.

In Chinese medical theory there are two categories of disharmonies which may result in insomnia. First are the deficiency patterns which have insomnia as one of the presenting complaints. Unlike the Qi deficiency associated with the pain and fatigue components of fibromyalgia syndrome, most of the deficiency patterns associated with sleep problems are deficiency of Blood or deficiency of Yin. There are several sub-categories which can be explored by the practitioner, and these will be covered in Chapter 5 (See Table 10c.)

There is also a group of excess patterns described by TCM which relate to sleep disorders. These are all "heat" or "fire" patterns, and while there is a possibility of one of them occurring in a fibromyalgia client, the deficiency patterns are much more consistent with the overall presentation, and should be considered first.

Secondary Signs and Symptoms

1. *Anxiety and/or depression*

Continuous physical discomfort coupled with unrelenting fatigue is a perfect formula to create depression, and it is extremely common among fibromyalgia and chronic fatigue clients. Anxiety or a wound-up agitated feeling inside is typical of Qi stagnation. Depression is a broader category and may accompany any deficiency pattern, but especially deficiency of Kidney, Lung, Spleen, or Heart Qi, or stagnation of Liver Qi. Depression is a part of many patterns. Other indicators such as pulse, tongue, Hara evaluation and questioning the client yield information to narrow the assessment. It is helpful to monitor a client's subjective reporting of mood as a means of observing positive change over time.

2. *Digestive Disturbances*

In classical TCM, digestive problems usually are related to deficiency of Spleen Qi, deficiency of Stomach Qi, stagnant Liver Qi or combinations. When the Spleen and/or Stomach is weak, the client can experience fatigue, muscular weakness, weak appetite, nausea, abdominal distension after eating, or loose stools. Stagnant Liver Qi will lead to distension, constipation or difficult elimination. Presence of the "Damp Pathogen" will also lead to indigestion, heartburn, loss of appetite, and feelings of distension or oppression in the chest, epigastric, and hypochondriac areas.

3. *Urinary Tract Problems*

This includes tendency toward bladder infections, incontinence, and bladder ptosis or dropping. These all have at their root a pattern of Qi deficiency; two of the functions of Qi are protection from invading disease entities, and holding the organs and tissues in their correct positions. Thus, deficiency of Qi may lead to this group of symptoms in some clients.

4. *Memory and Cognitive Difficulties*

Symptoms include memory impairment, inability to focus attention, inability to concentrate, slow processing of verbal instructions, slow internal thinking processes, inability to plan or think about future events, obsessive thinking patterns, and dulled responsiveness to incoming stimuli. "Fuzzy Headed" and "Fibro-fog" are terms people sometimes use to describe their cognitive impairment. Many clients claim this symptom is the most disturbing to their lifestyle, employment, and self-concept.

In Chinese medicine, language, memory, logic, dreaming, memory and planning are functions of Shen, which is housed in the Heart. The cognitive symptoms in fibromyalgia can arise from Heart deficiency patterns, typically deficient Heart Qi, deficient Heart Blood, or a combination. Once the capacity for cognition is established by the Heart, it is ruled by the Spleen, meaning the Spleen is responsible for smooth execution of the processes of cognition. Thus Spleen deficiency may also be a significant contributor to mental difficulties in fibromyalgia clients. Check pulse, tongue, or Hara to distinguish.

Chapter 5

Assessment and Pattern Differentiation for Fibromyalgia and Chronic Fatigue Syndromes

INITIAL INTERVIEW AND DATA COLLECTION

The first step in effectively treating people with fibromyalgia or chronic fatigue syndrome is to take a thorough history. Complete and accurate data is essential for treating any health challenge, but these syndromes have many variations and subtleties of presentation and degrees of severity. For best results it is crucial to treat each person individually. It is easy to fall into the therapeutic trap of treating the label "fibromyalgia syndrome" or "chronic fatigue" with point recipes or standard protocols rather than treating the individual human being who is seeking assistance.

The practitioner should allow sufficient time to interview the new client, perhaps as much as thirty to forty minutes during the first visit. It is highly recommended that a verbal interview be conducted even if a standard intake form is used in the clinic. It is important to take detailed notes for the person's file. It is helpful to ask a new client to prepare a written summary of her health history including accidents, illness, surgeries, pregnancies and significant emotional traumas, and bring it to the first session. This causes the client to review her personal history and organize it in a way that patterns may be more easily observed.

Many individuals with fibromyalgia or chronic fatigue have been to numerous doctors and other practitioners before seeking help through Asian therapies. Many have had unpleasant experiences with doctors who do not believe these conditions are "real, physical" disorders, and who have nothing new to offer the person to help their condition. Doctors can sometimes become frustrated with these people because the conditions are difficult to treat and most of the clients have sensitivities to medications. For many of the people who come for acutherapy, it may be the first time anyone has explored their situation in such depth. This attention to detail serves as a convincer of the practitioner's sincerity and competency.

In the practice of Chinese medicine assessment is accomplished by collecting data in four sensory categories: Looking, Listening, Asking, and

Palpation (Kaptchuk, 1983). This is a useful way of organizing complex histories and observations. A survey of potentially useful distinctions and questions in each category is given below, along with interpretative notes. The beginning practitioner is urged to consult standard books on Chinese medical theory for additional ideas for interpretation. The looking and listening sections are conducted by simple observation during the course of the interview, allowing the client to act as naturally as possible. In the following sections we will review a number of the signs and symptoms to look for during the intake interview.

Client Interview Part I: Looking

Complexion Color

Pale, Pink, Red, Sallow, Dark, Purplish?
Pale complexion suggests deficiency of Qi, Blood or Both.
Red or pink show presence of pernicious Heat pathogen or empty Heat.
Dark or Purplish suggest stagnation pattern.

General Build

Tall, Short, Heavy, Thin, Medium?
Constitutional patterns: Tall & Thin is more Yin; Short and Compact is
    more Yang. Underweight is more Yang, and obesity is more Yin.

Movement

Slow, rapid, easy, difficult; gestures; smooth or awkward gait?
A graceful, smooth gait and movement is a sign of abundant Qi and Blood flowing smoothly. Difficult, awkward, ponderous, or restricted movement may suggest stagnation in the muscles or joints affected, or overall stagnation or excess condition.

Affect

Lively, spirited, demonstrative, listless, sluggish?
According to Chinese medicine, a lively spirit and positive attitude are very positive signs that the patient will recover. Depression, sluggishness, and lack of affect are seen as negative signs. Affect relates closely to the Shen, or spirit. Continue to observe the client's affect even after the intake and in subsequent sessions. Some people are in the habit of "putting on their happy face" when they meet new people. It may take some time for the person to relax enough to put down her protective armor and let the true affect be observed.

Posture

Erect, balanced, stooped, bent?
Structural imbalances can be congenital, can be caused by muscular imbalances, habitual postures or activities, can be an adaptation to pain syndromes, or can be adaptation to organ dysfunction.

Tongue

Pale, red, purplish, dry, wet, teeth marks along edge?
Observation of the tongue is a classical Chinese diagnostic approach which can be studied and applied in astonishing depth and detail.   The practitioner is recommended to refer to texts which deal with the subject exhaustively (Maciocia, 1987).

Client Interview Part II: Listening

Voice Quality

Loud, gravely, quiet, soft, hoarse, moaning, whining
Chinese 5-Element energetics describes sounds which are related to each of the five energetic transformations (see Table 8). A soft or quiet voice, or dislike of speaking relates to Lung deficiency, and a loud, hoarse, or gravely voice relates to a Lung excess, such as Heat or Phlegm condition.

Diagnostic Sounds

Coughing, wheezing, sniffling, stomach growling, joints popping, sighing, clearing throat, inappropriate laughter or giggling, talkative. Noticing spontaneous sounds is helpful in determining organ problems in many cases.   Cough, wheeze, sniffles will relate mostly to Lung disharmonies; stomach or bowel sounds relate to Spleen or Stomach disharmonies.

Breath Pattern

The practitioner should note the relationship of the inhalation and exhalation parts of the breath cycle. Inhalation relates to Yin and increases the Water energy in the body, and exhalation relates to Yang and increases Fire energy in the body. These should be of equal strength, length, and depth to facilitate healthy energetic balance in the body. If one phase is stronger than the other, then corrective breathing exercises can be initiated by the practitioner. Practice at home by the client can improve the balance.

Client Interview Part III: Asking

In this part of the interview the practitioner asks questions about the client's problems, symptoms, history, and expectations of therapy.   Each question should be covered one-by-one. Make notes for the client's file. Appendix 1 is an intake form which includes these questions. It may be copied and used by owners of this book.

Chief complaint

Secondary complaints

How long ago was the onset?

Sudden or gradual onset?

Circumstances of onset

Examples: after an accident, childbirth, death in the family, surgery or other intervention, etc.

Head symptoms

Sinus, ears ringing, throat, eyes, headache, neck pain, vision

Chest symptoms

Palpitations, cough, mucus, catches colds easily, cardiac problems, asthma, respiratory allergies?

Digestion

Nausea, distension, ulcers, gas or bloating, diarrhea, constipation, sluggish digestion, irritable bowel, frequency of elimination?

Urinary

Frequency of urination, pale or dark urine, infections, burning, incontinence, bladder dropping, kidney stones, low back pain?

Female

Age of first menses, ease of menstruation, regularity of menstruation, PMS, pregnancies, (how many, how long ago, and ease of pregnancy and delivery), menopause?

Male

Prostate, GI tract problems? Discomfort on urination, incomplete urination, frequent or night-time urination?

Skin and Nails

Dry, moist, irritable, itchy, rashes, bruises, brittle nails, varicose veins? The skin reflects the health of the Lungs and Metal element. The nails reflect the vitality of the Liver, especially Liver Blood.

Musculo-skeletal

Presence or absence of pain, quality of pain, location of pain, duration of pain, continuous or intermittent, things which aggravate or diminish pain; muscles, joints, or both? (Have the client prepare a body map indicating the problem areas, and after the client lies down on the treatment table do a pressure pain map as well)

Sleep

Hours per night, quality, difficulty falling asleep, waking in the night, time of waking, feeling restored in the morning, difficulty rising?

Temperature

Tendency to chills or cold limbs, tendency to feel hot all over or in extremities? Hot flashes? Night sweats?

Psychological

What are the dominant emotions? Are any of the following commonly experienced by the client: depression, anxiety, dreams, memory, concentration, ease of planning, decision making, and self-motivation.

Medical History

Accidents (especially spinal and coccyx) or injuries; surgeries; significant childhood illnesses, use of maintenance medication? Did any of these occur just before or at the time of onset of fibromyalgia or chronic fatigue syndrome?

Previous Therapy

What therapies and self-help remedies has the client tried in the past and what helped or aggravated their condition? What self-directed therapies have they tried? Would they be willing to explore additional modalities or self-directed therapy such as exercise, nutrition, meditation and such? Would they like for you to recommend a book or a class on any of these subjects?

Expectations of Present Therapy

Explore the client's health goals, reasons for choosing the practitioner and modalities of therapy, and how their previous experience has contributed to their expectations. Some people are searching for miraculous cures which may not be realistic. Others have given up and expect very little from therapy. It is important to assist the client to have positive yet realistic expectations for her particular situation.

Client Interview Part IV: Body Mapping

Give the client color markers and a drawing of a human form, showing front, back and side views (Diagram 3, next page, may be copied and used by owners of this book). Ask them to color the areas on the drawing which correspond to their problem areas. Suggest that they color-code the areas according to severity, importance, consistency, or any criteria which is most relevant for them. Encourage them to describe what is going on as they color. Annotate the drawing using the client's words to describe what the colored areas indicate. Be sure to show the locations of surgical scars or trauma sites.

The use of a chart which the client colors is very helpful. The quality of data is usually very high, and it assists the client to clarify her/his experience. While many clients are very clear about which areas do or don't hurt, some clients become so overwhelmed by their condition that they lose the ability to make meaningful distinctions about their experience, which is a dis-empowering state. They may say "EVERYthing hurts" or "I can't do ANYthing". Part of the healing process for many is gaining better clarity and understanding of their body and their condition and move out of the pattern of grandiose generalizations.

The chart is also helpful as the course of therapy proceeds, because therapist and client can review it from time to time, noting how various areas have changed in location or intensity or quality of sensation. Ask the client to color another chart after a number of sessions; this assists the client in reviewing her/his progress over the weeks and provides a visual map of change.

Client Interview Part V: Palpation

Tender Point Exam

Frequently people who have not been medically diagnosed with fibromyalgia syndrome may come for assistance from an oriental bodywork therapist, massage therapist, or acupuncturist. While it is not appropriate for these practitioners to render a medical diagnosis, it is certainly appropriate and helpful to test the tender point areas when fibromyalgia is suspected. Refer to the tender point diagram in Chapter 1.

The classical tender points closely correspond to several of the major acupoints in the body as follows: (Each is bilateral).

Gall Bladder-20	(occipital margin)
Stomach-9	(C-5 to C-7, scalenes)
Gall Bladder-21	(top of trapezius)
Triple Burner-15	(supraspinatus)
Kidney 27	(sterno-clavicular junction)
Large Intestine-10 and -11	(lateral epicondyle)
Gall Bladder-30	(greater trochanter)
Namikoshi's point	
halfway between	
GB-30 and GB-26	(gluteus medius)
Liver-8	(knee)

Pulses

Chinese pulse assessment can be very helpful in deciding how to treat the condition (Zhen,1981; Kaptchuk,1983). The major distinctions are:

Weak   vs.   Forceful
Slow   vs.   Rapid
Deep   vs.   Superficial
Choppy, rough, wiry, tight, or slippery
Right side or left side stronger
Any of the 5-Elements sites especially weak or forceful

While it is beyond the scope of this text to give an in-depth discussion of Chinese pulse diagnosis, it is well worth learning. Most practitioners can make simple distinctions in pulses with a little practice. It is recommended that practitioners find a teacher for advanced study in pulse assessment.

Practitioners who are familiar with the Five Elements approach already have an elegant model for organizing signs and symptoms. The practitioner can compare his/her findings, along with lists of symptoms, with the listings in Table 8. There are several good books on the subject, but guidance from an advanced teacher of Chinese Medicine will be valuable to the serious student.

Therapist body mapping

Next prepare a body map of pressure pain areas. Focus mostly on the areas where the client subjectively experiences discomfort, and on related areas. Also focus on the classical assessment areas for Chinese medicine such as the Back Shu Points and the Hara. There will usually be soreness, tightness, or sensitivity to pressure at the classical diagnostic points. This helps guide the practitioner in determining which specific patterns are most probable. There are many good descriptions and maps of the diagnostic points in the acupuncture and acupressure textbooks.

Use a clean body outline chart, and indicate findings with color-coding or with a numbering system. Color-coding is an excellent method to mark tissue quality. A numbering system from one to five can be used to indicated the client's subjective experience of pressure pain. Most therapists will develop a personal system which can be used quickly and which captures the information for assessment purposes, and to compare changes over a series of sessions.

Meridian Palpation

Using the client's verbal reporting and colored chart as guides, the practitioner can gently explore the painful areas to differentiate which of the meridian pathways and points are most involved. This is another procedure which may assist the client in making distinctions about the areas that are most involved and the ones which are less severely affected or not affected. While palpating the affected channels the therapist may also check key points such as the source points, accumulation points, tonification points, and sedation points for reactivity.

Meridians which are reactive along much of their length or have sensitivity in key points will be especially important in the treatment strategy, as they are locations of stagnation. The reader may refer to Tables 10a, 10b, 10c, Table 11, and Table 12 for acupoint indications for fibromyalgia and chronic fatigue.

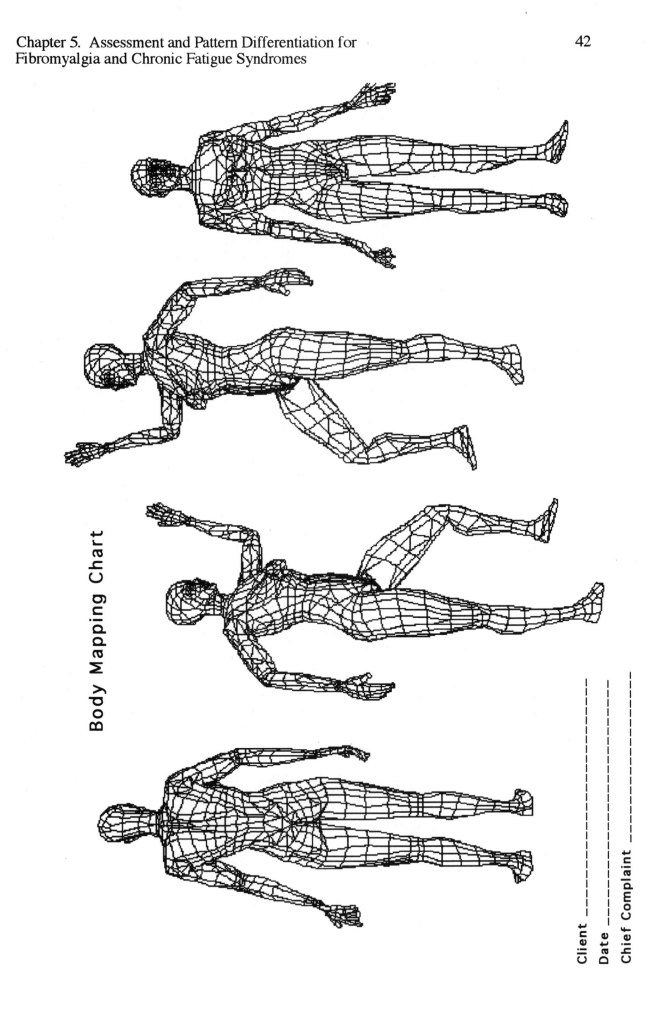

Body Mapping Chart

Client _____

Date _____

Chief Complaint _____

Table 8. Common Assessment Characteristics and Five Elements

Characteristic	Water	Wood	Fire	Earth	Metal
Colors	Blue, black	Green	Red, pink	Yellow, tan	White
Voice Quality	Moaning	Shouting	Laughter	Sing-song	Whining
Body Type	Ectomorph	Mesomorpth	Endomorph	Endomorph	Ectomorph
Unbalanced Emotions	Fearful, timid Non-assertive Overwhelm	Angry, frustrated Irritable	Bitter, Unforgiving Hateful	Worrisome Obsessive	Sad, Remorseful Can't let go
Balanced Emotions	Will Power	Patience	Joy, Enthusiasm	Confidence	Contentment
Healing Activity	Qi Gong Tai Chi Standing Postures	Yoga, Stretching, Range-of-Motion	Aerobic Exercise; Walking, Swimming	Sitting Meditation	Yoga in Lying Postures, Breath work
Tissues Governed	Bones	Ligaments Tendons	Blood Vessels	Muscles Fascia	Skin
Organs and Meridians	Kidneys Bladder	Liver Gall Bladder	Heart Sm.Intestine	Spleen Pancreas Stomach	Lungs Large Intestine
Joints	Knees, Lumbar, Ankles	Shoulders Neck	Elbows	Hips	Wrists
Tongue Region	Back	Edges	Tip	Center	Behind tip
Bodywork Styles Best Suited	Cranio-Sacral	Deep Tissue Joint Mobilization	Circulatory Massage	Lymphatic Drainage	Visceral Hara work
Body Fluids	Urine	Tears	Sweat	Saliva	Nasal mucus
Sense	Hearing	Vision	Hearing	Taste	Smell
Pulse Quality	Sinking	Wiry	Rapid	Slippery	Floating
Climate	Cold	Wind	Heat	Dampness	Dry
Diagnostic Sounds	Yawning	Sighing, Clearing Throat	Hiccups Giggling	Stomach Growling Belching	Cough Wheeze Sniffles

INTERPRETATION OF ASSESSMENT DATA

Once the interview and examination process is completed, it is necessary to organize the information into a meaningful and useful preliminary assessment. In Chinese medicine, every assessment is a hypothesis and every treatment is an experiment designed to test the hypothesis. Human beings are complex organisms which present dozens of discernible signs and symptoms. From this milieu it is necessary to make clinical sense so that the most appropriate treatment may be given. It is also necessary to check key pieces of data on subsequent visits, because when therapy is very effective and/or the client is making lifestyle changes, the clinical picture can change from session to session. There are often many layers of disharmony in fibromyalgia and chronic fatigue, and the therapist and client must explore each layer as it reveals itself over the course of treatments. Table 9 summarizes symptoms according to three of the most widely used TCM models.

For most practitioners of acupuncture or oriental bodywork therapy it will be most helpful to start at the level of Qi and Blood, Yin and Yang, for their fibromyalgia clients. Having collected the interview and examination data, compare the prominent signs and symptoms with the listings in Table 10 a, b, and c. At the far right in Table 10 are listings of acupoints which may be used to help balance the disharmony. For the serious student, specific patterns are listed under each major heading. The patterns are explored in depth in many acupuncture texts (See Maciocia 1989). A few of the most common ones which relate to fibromyalgia and chronic fatigue are briefly discussed below.

COMMON PATTERNS OF DISHARMONY

Vital Substances and Zang Fu Patterns

Generalized Qi Deficiency

Qi deficiency is characterized by dislike of movement and activity, fatigue or tiredness, weak immune system (easily catches colds, chronic infections, allergies, etc.), poor quality of metabolic processes in the body (weak digestion or absorption, poor blood oxygenation, weak thyroid, blood-sugar imbalances, etc.), and organs and/or substances failing to stay in their proper places (varicose veins, haemorrhoids, bladder or uterus ptosis, incontinence, easy bruising, etc.). For fibromyalgia and chronic fatigue, the most common type of Qi deficiency is Spleen Qi deficiency, which leads to Dampness.

Spleen Qi Deficiency

In Chinese medicine the Spleen has functions which include transportation and transformation of fluids, ruling the muscles, and serving as the "root of post-heaven Qi. Several of the main symptoms of fibromyalgia and chronic fatigue relate to impairment of these functions. Lymphatic accumulation or sluggishness, muscle pain, and fatigue correlate with these functions, respectively. When the Spleen becomes weakened, it cannot perform its function of transportation and transformation efficiently, and

Dampness accumulates. This is closely correlated with the muscular pain, weakness, and abnormal texture of the muscle tissue found in fibromyalgia.

Fatigue relates to the Spleen (and Stomach) role as "root of post-heaven Qi" in that the digestive process is inefficient and the person is not extracting the Qi from the food, or perhaps the food is processed and lacking in Qi. Digestive disturbances can include anorexia, loose stools and abdominal distension and irritable bowel. In Chinese medicine, most of the digestive functions are associated with the Spleen rather than the intestines, so intestinal problems are usually treated with points on the Spleen meridian.

Weakness of the limbs, lassitude, edema, sallow complexion, excessive worry, and mental exhaustion are part of the pattern as well. Fuzzy-headedness, inability to focus or concentrate, and feeling of a "pressure band" around the head also indicate the presence of the Damp pathogen, which easily accumulates when Spleen Qi is deficient.

The primary causes of Spleen Qi deficiency are improper diet and excessive worry and mental work. Dietary factors which especially damage Spleen Qi include cold, raw, and wet foods, excessive sugar intake, and artificial sweeteners. Overeating also stresses the Spleen and its partner, the Stomach.

Generalized Blood Deficiency

Blood deficiency is characterized by anemia, dizziness, disturbances in the body's cyclical activities (sleep cycle, menstrual cycle, hunger cycle, thirst cycle, etc.), tremors, emaciation, and numbness in extremities.

Liver Qi Stagnation

Depression, melancholy, feeling "wound up", painful menstruation, distension or pain under the ribs, spontaneous sighing, breast tenderness, fibroid tumors in breasts or uterus, mood swings, belching, diarrhea, and growling or churning stomach are all symptoms of Liver Qi Stagnation.

Practitioners of oriental medicine usually work with several different models, including Five Elements, Zang-Fu, Vital Substances, Eight Principles and Meridian theory. This makes it possible to look at illness through several different lenses. Many times a particular client's presentation will fit very well into one model, but not into others. Table 9 gives suggestions for interpreting common fibromyalgia and chronic fatigue symptoms through three different models.

Pernicious Influences

Maciocia (1994) describes chronic fatigue (myalgic encephalitis, ME) as invasion of Pernicious Wind which is never cleared and converts to Heat, Phlegm -Heat or Damp-Heat inside the body. This weakens Qi and/or Yin, leading to a downward spiral in the condition. Maciocia suggests that use of antibiotic and immunization is a cause for the body's failure to eliminate pathogenic factors. He states that every case of ME exhibits a pattern of deficiency (Qi, Yang, or Yin) with an excess pattern, usually Dampness.

Table 9. Common Symptoms of Fibromyalgia and Chronic Fatigue and the Models of Chinese Medicine

Symptom	Zang Fu Patterns	Five Element Patterns	Vital Substances & Pernicious
Fatigue or exhaustion	Kidney, Spleen, Lung	Water, Earth, Metal	Qi deficient Yang or Yin deficient
Headaches	Liver, Gall Bladder	Wood	Blood or Qi stagnant
Short term memory loss	Heart, Kidney, Spleen	Fire, Earth	Blood deficient Dampness
Widespread muscle pain	Liver, Kidney, Spleen	Earth	Qi stagnant; channel obstructions, Damp
Difficulty concentrating	Heart, Spleen	Earth	Blood deficient
Joint pain	Liver, Kidney, Spleen	Wood	Qi/Blood stag; Dampness, Cold.
Lymph Node Pain	Spleen	Earth	Blood
Sore Throat	Lung	Metal	Yin deficient
Fever or sensation of fever	Lung, Stomach	Fire	Yin deficient. or Heat excess
Blurry vision	Liver	Wood	Blood deficient
Depression	Kidney, Heart, Liver	Wood, Water, Fire	Shen, Qi stagnation
Insomnia	Kidney	Fire, Water	Yin deficient
Abdominal pain/ distension	Spleen, Liver	Earth, Wood	Dampness
Scratchy or dry eyes	Liver	Wood	False Heat
Numb/tingling extremities	Liver, Kidneys	Wood, Water	Blood deficient
Allergies	Spleen, Lung	Earth, Metal	Wind Heat, Wind Cold
Heart palpitations	Heart	Fire	Qi or Blood deficient
Night sweats	Heart	Fire	Yin deficient
Constipation	Liver, Kidney Stomach	Earth, Wood	Yin or Yang deficient
Irritable bowel syndrome	Liver, Spleen	Metal, Earth	Qi, Blood stagnation
Muscular weakness	Spleen	Earth	Qi deficient
Dizziness, vertigo	Liver, Gall Bladder	Wood	Wind
Panic attacks; anxiety	Heart	Fire	Shen, Heat
Chemical sensitivities	Liver	Wood	Qi Stagnation

Five Element and Zang Fu Patterns

The most common Five Element disharmony for fibromyalgia is "deficient Earth " with "excess Wood", leading to the pattern "Liver invading Spleen". Earth element includes Spleen and Stomach and rules the muscles. Disharmony of Earth can lead to muscular complaints, especially those associated with Damp conditions, as Dampness is the climatic factor associated with Earth. Fatigue and depression are frequently associated with the Wood element which includes Liver and Gall Bladder. Fatigue can also indicate deficient Water or Earth.

Zang-Fu Patterns are useful for acutherapists and herbalists. They are covered very thoroughly in several textbooks of Chinese medicine, especially Maciocia (1989) and Ross (1985) Table 10 a, b, and c show common patterns found in chronic fatigue and fibromyalgia. Assessment and treatment information is given along with acupoints or body areas to palpate; tenderness in these regions helps confirm assessment. Table 10 a. shows patterns with fatigue as a main symptom, Table 10 b. deals with muscle pain, and Table 10 c. shows patterns related to sleep problems.

Table 10 a. Main Zang-Fu Patterns Leading to FATIGUE

Main TCM Patterns	Key Symptoms	Pulse	Tongue	Point Palpation	Treatment Points
Spleen Qi or Spleen Yang Deficient	Poor appetite, epigastric discomfort, muscular weakness, irritable digestion	Empty	Pale, wet, puffy, with tooth imprints	SP-3, SP-4, SP-6, SP-9, Umbilicus	SP-2, SP-3, Ren-12, Liv-13, BL-20, BL-21 Moxa
Lung Qi or Lung Yang Deficient	Breathless, quiet voice, catches cold easily, cough, spontaneous sweat, dry or sore throat	Weak Empty	Pale	Lu-1 & 2 Lu-3 & 4 Lu-5, Lu-7, Lu-9, BL-13 Ileocecal valve	Lu-9, Lu-7 ST-36, Ren-6 Ren-17, BL-43, DU-12, BL-13 Moxa
Kidney Yang Deficient	Extreme fatigue, depression, sore low back & knees, freq. pale urine, feels cold weak libido, impotence	Deep, Slow Weak	pale swollen	Lumbar Lower belly Ki-3 Ki-6 BL-23	Ki-3, Ki-7 Ren-4 Sp-6 BL-23 DU-4, Moxa

Table 10 b. Main Zang-Fu Patterns Leading to MUSCLE PAIN

Main TCM Patterns	Key Symptoms	Pulse	Tongue	Point Palpation	Treatment Points
Dampness or Damp-Heat in the Muscles	Aches, fatigue, heavy feeling in head or body, dull headache, memory problems, "foggy" thinking, lack of stamina, pressure in chest or epigastrum	Soggy Slippery; If Heat is present, pulse will also be Rapid	Sticky white coating = Damp. Yellow tongue coat = Heat	Spleen, gallbladder, and kidney channels, SCM musc. SP-9, SP-10, ST-40, skin feels moist	SP-9, SP-6, SP-3, TB-7, BL-20, BL-22, Ren-12, Ren-9, LI-11, TB-5, DU-14 No Moxa if Heat Present
Liver Qi Stagnation	Tired in afternoon, depression, tight in ribs or chest, sighing, belching, poor appetite, wound-up feeling, PMS, breasts tender, irritability	Wiry	Normal color or red along sides or slightly purplish	Rib margins, intercostal muscles, mid-back tight or sore, Liv-3, Liv-14, Sp-6	GB-34, Liv-3, Liv-13, TB-3, Liv-14, Sp-6, BL-18

Table 10 c. Main Zang-Fu Patterns for SLEEP DISTURBANCE

Main TCM Patterns	Key Symptoms	Pulse	Tongue	Point Palpation	Treatment Points
Heart Blood Deficient	Difficulty falling asleep, but sleeps well after falling asleep; palpitations, depression, dizzy	Empty, choppy, or thin	Pale, may have midline crack at tip	Sternum, Ren-14, BL-14-15	Ht-5, PC-6, BL-15, Ren-6 Ren-14, Ren-15, Ht-7, St-36, Sp-6
Kidney Yin Deficient	Wakes up often during night; lack of will power, weak knees/legs, tinnitis, dry mouth, night sweats	Floating-empty or Rapid-fine	Red without coating	Lumbar, Knees, ankles, lower abdomen	Ki-3, Ren-4, Lu-7+Ki-6, Sp-6, BL-23, BL-52
Liver-Fire or Heart Fire	Dream-disturbed sleep, Sleepwalking, irritability, dizziness, dry throat, dry eyes	Floating-empty	Red without coating	Rib margins, intercostal muscles, mid back, sternum	Liv-8, Liv-3, Liv-14, Ren-4, Sp-6, P-7, Du-24, GB-15, BL-47, Ki-6, Ht-8,
Gall Bladder Deficiency	Wakes up very early in morning and cannot go back to sleep; sighing, timidity, lack of courage, blurry vision, nervous	Weak	Pale or normal	Right rib margins, Gallbladder meridian, GB-30, GB-40	GB-40, GB-38, GB-30, Liv-3

Vital Substances

Frequently it is difficult to arrive at an exact assessment with complex clients. Determining whether Yin or Yang, Qi or Blood is the most significant part of the person's patterns is an excellent assessment; it is not necessary or always relevant to identify which Organ is most deficient. Table 11 summarizes assessment information and principle treatment points for patterns of the Vital Substances. Under each pattern, the specific Organ patterns which may be included are listed.

Summary

It is entirely possible for a person to manifest more than one of these patterns simultaneously or to move through several of them over time as their health status changes. For the beginning oriental bodywork therapist, the overriding consideration will be to give an overall tonifying treatment, which will boost the client's Qi and get it moving, to assist her with relaxation and pain minimization. The next goal is to clear the Damp pathogen, which will reduce the muscular symptoms and the fuzzy-headed feeling. As the therapist continues to learn and fine-tune diagnostic skills, she can begin to incorporate more specifically targeted treatments strategies.

Table 11. Vital Substance Patterns in Fibromyalgia and Chronic Fatigue

Pattern	Signs & Symptoms	Pulse	Tongue	Acupoints

Qi Deficiency
    Spleen Qi Deficient
    Heart Qi Deficient
    Lung Qi Deficient
    Stomach Qi Deficient
	Tired, fatigue; vague achy pain, migrating pain, muscular weakness, listless, depression, bright-pale complexion, low immunity. May also have: no appetite, heart palpitations on exertion, weak voice, breathless, cough, loose stools, abdominal distension	Empty Weak	Pale or normal color	St-36, SP-6 LIE-4, LI-11 Ren-6, Ki-3 BL-23, Sp-3 Lu-9, Lu-7, Ren-6, Du-14, Ren-12, Back-Shu Points

Yang Deficiency
    Spleen Yang Deficient
    Kidney Yang Deficient
    Heart Yang Deficient
	Any symptoms of Qi deficiency plus: cold extremities, chilly body, extreme exhaustion, impotence, abundant clear urination, apathy, edema, fluid retention	Deep Slow Weak	Pale, wet, puffy, swollen	Points for Qi deficiency plus: Du-4, Ren-8, Du-14, Ren-4, Du-20, BL-23, Ren-17 Use Moxa

Blood Deficiency
    Heart Blood Deficient
    Liver Blood Deficient
	Dizziness, fuzzy thinking, insomnia, numbness in limbs, pale lips, dull-pale complexion. May also exhibit poor ability to plan, poor memory, anxiety, easily startled, difficulty concentrating, restless, palpitations without exertion, scanty menstruation, muscle cramps and spasms,	Choppy	Pale and dry or withered	Sp-3, Sp-6, Sp-10, BL-17, Liv-8, Ht-7, PC-6, BL-18, St-36, Ren-4, Sp-8, Ren-6

Yin Deficiency
    Kidney Yin Deficient
    Heart Yin Deficient
    Lung Yin Deficient
    Stomach Yin Deficient
	Any signs of deficient Blood plus: extreme exhaustion, feeling of heat in body, "burned-out", night sweats, hot flashes, hot hands-feet-chest, malar flush, extreme thirst, low-grade fever in afternoon or evening	Floating	Thin, dry, withered, cracks on surface	Points for deficient Blood plus: Ht-6 + Ki-7, Ki-6 + Lu-7, Ren-4, Ren-6, Lu-9, Ki-3; Moxa prohibited

Qi Stagnation Liver Qi Stagnation	Irritability, depression, abdominal distension, bloating, sighing, nausea, hiccuping, reflux, belching, indigestion,	Wiry tight	normal or purplish	GB-34, Liv-3, Liv-8, Liv-14, BL-18, GB-41, PC-6, Liv-13, Du-20

Blood Stagnation
    Stagnant Liver Blood
    Stagnant Heart Blood
	Sharp or stabbing pain, severe menstrual cramps, lumps, masses, fibroids, severe headaches, tightness or feeling of pressure in chest or abdomen	Choppy, full, wiry	Dark purple	LI-11, Sp-6, Sp-4, Sp-8, Liv-13, BL-60, St-30, PC-6, Liv-2, Liv-3, Liv-8, Sp-10

Chapter 6

Treatment Principles and Methods

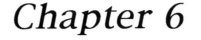
Treat Both Root & symptoms from the beginning

TREATING THE "ROOT" AND THE "BRANCHES"

After assessment data is collected and organized the therapist has a basis for beginning to treat a client with chronic fatigue or fibromyalgia. Chinese medicine distinguishes between treatment of the "root" and treatment of the "branches" or symptoms. In most cases the practitioner will choose to treat both root and symptoms from the beginning. Treating only the root-cause imbalance will ultimately lead to improvement of the symptoms, but it is also true that lessening the symptoms early will release stagnant energy needed for healing, increase the trust and rapport between client and practitioner, and boost the morale, stamina and motivation of the client. The best results come when the client is motivated to get involved with lifestyle modification such as exercise, meditation or nutritional changes. Lessening the muscular pain and boosting the energy make it more possible for the client to do these things.

New clients usually expect to feel better after only one or two sessions, so it is important to provide pain relief, energy boosting, and other desirable benefits right away. It is important to educate clients that natural and holistic therapies work with the body's own healing energies, that healing is a process which occurs gradually, layer-by-layer, and regular sessions are very important. The wise therapist will also make suggestions of simple things (acupoints to work, easy stretches, a breathing exercise) that clients can do at home, any time, with ease, so they can begin to take back their autonomy and independence.

self therapies

COURSE OF TREATMENTS
AND WHAT TO EXPECT

In the early stages of treatment (the first six to twelve weeks), it is recommended that the client receive at least one session per week, if possible. These may be from thirty to ninety minutes, depending on the client's ability to receive acupuncture or bodywork, financial concerns, and scheduling factors. If the assessment is accurate, and the practitioner efficient and experienced, one session per week of acupuncture or oriental bodywork will make an excellent beginning. If it is within the financial means and scheduling possibilities for the client, then two visits per week could be recommended for the first few weeks. If a client can only afford to come every two or three weeks initially, that is better than no therapy, but progress will be slower. In these cases, it is crucial to teach the client self-therapy to do at home.

After the initial period, treatments can be spaced further apart, such as every ten to fourteen days. As the beneficial effects of the treatments last longer and the client learns more self-care techniques and lifestyle changes, practitioner and client can decide upon an appropriate schedule. Many clients can eventually establish a maintenance schedule of one session per month, with perhaps an extra session or two in the case of a flare-up of symptoms, or during times of increased stress. Some individuals will want to maintain a weekly schedule, but many will appreciate having their sessions at longer intervals. Ideally the schedule should meet the client's needs both therapeutically and financially.

Regularity of sessions is extremely important. Many of the factors which are correlated with the onset of fibromyalgia syndrome have an element of irregularity and unpredictability inherent in them. As a part of re-training the body systems, it cannot be over-emphasized that the client needs to have regular sessions. The practitioner should strongly recommend incorporating regularity into other aspects of the lifestyle as well, such as meal times, sleep times, exercise time, work schedule, and so on. It is easy for the fibromyalgia client to feel overwhelmed, so these changes must be done gradually, one item at a time. For example, she could start by arising at the same time each morning and going to bed at the same time each night. After two to three weeks, she could add another change. The more the person can regain control of everyday activities, the better the outcome. If possible, other family members can be counselled to assist the client in these goals. The practitioner of Chinese medicine should think of himself/herself as a role model for clients and therefore should also practice living in harmony with the natural laws and developing self-mastery.

It is important to communicate to clients that excellent results can be obtained with Asian modalities. However, this will occur over time with ongoing treatments, as chronic deficiency patterns and stagnation patterns take time to improve. There is no "quick fix". The results may be amplified or decreased by a client's willingness to explore stress management and lifestyle modification. The therapist should be prepared to offer multiple resources to assist the client exploring lifestyle changes.

Typically the client will experience lessening of some symptoms, including pain and low energy, for one to four days after a session in these early stages. Then the symptoms may tend to return. Some individuals will have a day or two of soreness after massage or bodywork, and other symptoms such as headache may increase as well. Fibromyalgia and chronic fatigue clients usually have toxins and metabolic waste products stored in the organs and muscles, and acupuncture or bodywork can allow the tissues to release them, causing soreness, headache, digestive disturbance and other symptoms. It is wise to start with gentle treatment to determine individual response. If there is little or no cleansing reaction, more vigorous treatment may be employed next session.

Gradually the relief should last longer as more sessions are completed. Occasionally a client does not improve as much as the practitioner would expect based on his experience with other chronic fatigue or fibromyalgia clients. When this happens, the practitioner can work with the individual to identify factors which may be blocking progress. Perhaps there is a chronic source of stress from the person's job, family, emotional issues, or other areas which needs to be handled to accomplish better improvement. In such situations, it may be appropriate to suggest mental health counselling when the individual is open to it.

Relapses

Relapses almost inevitably occur for chronic fatigue and fibromyalgia clients. As the person begins to feel better and have more energy, they often tend to resume the familiar pattern of over-doing things, and find themselves back in the same situations that started the problems in the first place. The practitioner should regard relapses not as a failure, but as a part of the learning process that must occur over time. It is important to teach this attitude to the client, so they can see their inevitable downfalls as a positive part of an overall progression toward better health and learn to identify the factors which may precipitate a relapse or flare.

Each time the person goes through a cycle of improvement followed by relapse, she refines her understanding of her lifestyle, stress, and emotional patterns as they affect her health. She learns to identify factors which can either bring on a relapse, or cause the condition to improve. On the bright side, most people tend to improve much more rapidly and easily each time they go through a relapse or "flare" of symptoms. During relapses it may be helpful to do an extra session or two until the person is once again in a stable improvement phase. It can be helpful if the client will keep a journal of health-related behaviors and activities, including foods, exercise, weather conditions, sleep, travel, work and family stresses, and other factors. Correlating these with overall well-being and specific symptoms can teach the person much that will be useful in managing chronic fatigue or fibromyalgia.

The First Four to Six Sessions   *"get things moving"*

Because fibromyalgia and chronic fatigue frequently involve numerous body systems and the symptoms are generalized within most clients, it is recommended that the practitioner start with the primary objective of "getting things moving." This may refer to Qi or Blood in the oriental approach, or to lymphatic fluids, circulatory blood, and neurological stimulation in the Western framework.

When working with hands-on oriental bodywork approaches (shiatsu, acupressure, tuina, anma, Jin Shin Do, etc.) the practitioner would ideally administer a full-body treatment in which every meridian pathway and each major muscle group and joint is stimulated in the course of the session. Abdominal (Hara) massage is essential, with emphasis on the lower right quadrant in the region of the ileo-caecal valve. The ileo-caecal valve is the sphincter muscle which controls the flow of digestive material from the small intestine to the large intestine. Like any other muscle, it can be hypertonic, hypotonic, or spastic. If the valve is too loose, diarrhea may be the result. If too tight, constipation may occur. A spastic valve can produce alternating constipation and diarrhea. Hara massage administered by the

abdominal massage / Hara is essential with emphasis on lower Right region of the ileo-ceecal valve.

therapist or by the client as homework is an important technique for alleviating digestive complaints.

The entire spine, sacrum and occipital areas are also extremely important to treat. These areas are rich in acupoints, meridian pathways, muscle attachments, and nerves. If the client is coming for short sessions it may take two or three visits to address all the meridians. The therapist must be flexible and open-minded, always giving first priority to the client's comfort and well-being.

Careful attention must be given to appropriate pressure application, especially for fibromyalgia clients. Techniques which are gentle yet vigorous, rhythmic, and stimulating must be employed, taking care to stay within the individual's physical comfort zone. Rocking, jostling, passive stretching, rubbing briskly with the whole hand, palm pressure, thumb pressure, hand-rolling, frictioning, and static pressure may all be employed. Many clients will be extremely sensitive in certain areas or over the entire body, so it is important to maintain verbal communication and coaching as needed throughout the sessions. The diagnostic tender points and other lymphatic reflex areas are especially likely to be pressure sensitive. Be prepared to change to a gentler technique any time the client requests it.

Some clients with fibromyalgia enjoy deep pressure, so be prepared to deliver that as well. Many clients cannot lie still in one position for more than a few minutes at a time, so allow them the opportunity to change positions when necessary. The therapist should be familiar with prone, supine, and lateral recumbent client positioning and techniques. Floor work (shiatsu) or table work are both appropriate, as long as the client can be relaxed and comfortable during the session. Before using a floor-work format, make sure the person can get down to the floor and up again, with minimal assistance. A full-body treatment regime for fibromyalgia is offered later in this text (Chapter 11). It can be used in its entirety or selected portions may be used for shorter sessions.

When treating with acupuncture, select points which address the patterns identified in assessment, and work with local and distal points to relieve pain. For example, if pain is worst in the neck and shoulders, local points such as GB-20, GB-21, LI-16, TB-15, SI-11 could be selected. Distal points such as GB-34, GB-40, LI-4, TB-5, and SI-4 would work well with these local points.

Later Treatments

It is important to continue to keep the energies and the fluids moving in the body. If stagnation or deficiency returns or increases, the client will experience an increase in stiffness, soreness, aching, and fatigue. After four to six sessions, it will be important to add points which address the particular imbalances which have been assessed in the client. Please note that the general treatment points given in the tables in this chapter will continue to be valuable all through the course of treatment, and can be taught to the client for home acupressure therapy.

If the assessment is not clear, continue to work in the more general way. As assessment skills improve, and the practitioner begins to more fully understand the energetics of the individual, it is appropriate to move to a more specific level of treatment. Source points, tonification points, and Back-Shu points for the deficient Organs become increasingly important at this time. Acupuncture texts have complete listing of the points used to treat the specific patterns of disharmony. Also refer to Tables 10 and 11 in Chapter 5.

Many clients improve greatly, and want to shift from a weekly schedule of treatments to a maintenance schedule of once per month or even longer between sessions. It is recommend to gradually increase the time between sessions to find the rhythm which works best for each individual.

VALUABLE CHANNELS AND ACUPOINTS FOR FIBROMYALGIA AND CHRONIC FATIGUE

Pain Therapy   *urinary Bladder, Large intestine, gall bladder*

Chapter 7 contains concepts and strategies for pain management. Three of the most important channels for relieving widespread body discomfort are the Urinary Bladder, Large Intestine, and the Gall Bladder pathways. Fibromyalgia muscle pain is related to accumulation of Dampness in the tissues, so points such as SP-9, SP-6, SP-3, ST-40, Ren-12, Ren-9, BL-22, LI-11, TB-7, LU-10, and DU-14 to expel Dampness. *combination GB-20, UB-10, GB-21, Li-16*

The combination of GB-20, UB-10, GB-21, and LI-16 releases much of the neck and upper-body discomfort. LI-4 and LI-11 are also valuable for generalized body discomfort. The Four Gates of Pain (Liver-3 and LI-4, bilateral) are very helpful for widespread pain from any cause. *Four gates of Pain bilateral Liver 3 L intestine 4*

The sternocleidomastoid muscle is usually hypertonic and extremely tender in these syndromes; treat it with gentle thumb pressure or gentle squeezing along its length. Hold gentle pressure on points which are especially tight or tender; in fibromyalgia clients this will usually be the mastoid end (insertion) of the muscle. Working gently with the sternocleidomastoid and with the suboccipital muscles can also help relieve intra-cranial pressure which contributes to the headaches and foggy thinking that are frequently associated with fibromyalgia. Needling is not recommended on the sternocleidomastoid.

Vigorous frictioning (as much pressure as the person can take) on the entire scalp, forehead, and behind the ears along the mastoid process is helpful for relieving head and neck discomfort. For lower-body discomfort, treating the sacrum and sacro-iliac joint, GB-30, Namikoshi's Extra Point, GB-31, GB-34, and UB-54 are very helpful. *scalp forehead & behind Ears (Vigorous) FRICTION*

Lower body discomfort - GB-30 namikoshi's Extra Point, GB-31 GB-34 UB-54.

Moxa can also be very beneficial for musculo-skeletal pain associated with fibromyalgia. When the individual finds direct pressure too uncomfortable, moxa is an excellent alternative to massage or acupressure in the early stages of therapy.

Fatigue *(gall bladder, spleen, + liver channels)*

ST 36 - SP 6 - LI 4, - Lu 7 - Ren - 4 - Ren - 6 - Ren 12 - Ren 17 - Du - 4

In an article on the use of oriental bodywork therapy for chronic fatigue syndrome the author (Young, 1993) emphasises the use of Gall Bladder, Spleen, and Liver channels. Valuable Qi-boosting points include ST-36, SP-6, LI-4, LU-7, Ren-4, Ren-6, Ren-12, Ren-17, and Du-4. When giving hands-on therapy, holding these points for several minutes each is indicated. Steady pressure will allow the points to "fill"; hold until a strong, steady therapeutic pulse is felt in the points for at least ten to twelve breath cycles. When using acupuncture needles to treat, use reinforcing technique on the Qi-boosting points.

indirect Moxa

Moxa is recommended for cold, weak or exhausted clients. If the pulse is slow, weak, and deep, and the tongue is pale, wet, or puffy, moxa is indicated. Indirect moxa can be applied to individual points or to larger areas such as the sacrum and Hara. If the skin is cool to the touch in these areas, consider spending the time it takes to do this treatment. Moxa can also be used at home by the client. Be sure to carefully instruct in it's use, and let the person practice in the office so you can see they are doing it correctly. If there are Heat signs, such as red tongue or rapid pulse, do not use moxa. Moxa is discussed more thoroughly below. In addition to acutherapy and massage for energy boosting, it is also wise to look at other modalities such as breath work, Qi Gong, Chinese herbal formulas, and nourishment. More will be said about these in a later chapter.

Do Not use if signs of Heat

Depression *HT-7, PC-6, Ren 17, Liv 3*

Acutherapy is an excellent modality for lifting the spirits. Once the energy is mobilized, the person will probably notice an improvement in mood almost immediately. There are several valuable acupoints which can be needled or massaged when depression is a major symptom. These include HT-7, PC-6, Ren-17, and LIV-3. Chinese herbal formulas can also be employed, as well as aromatherapy (see Chapter 10).

Sleep Disturbance *pc-6, Ht-7, DB-20, GV-16, UB-38, BV-24, 5, Ren-17, Ki-6, UB-62*

For people with fibromyalgia and chronic fatigue, inability to have consistent restorative sleep is one of the more difficult symptoms because it is so closely linked to how one feels. Energy level, depression and muscle discomfort improve when the person is able to get restful sleep. Medication is frequently prescribed, but long-term use of sleeping pills can add to health issues, including poor sleep quality. Acupressure can be done at home by the client or a family member, and with other strategies, can assist with improving sleep.

The client who has sleep problems will benefit by using several strategies together. Sleep habits can be considered a lifestyle choice in that the individual has choices about factors which contribute to good sleep. Aromatherapy and herbal teas have been mentioned in other parts of this book (Chapter 10). The individual should begin to make her sleep patterns as regular as possible. Regular times of going to bed and arising in the morning should be chosen so that seven to eight hours are allocated for sleep, more if possible while recovering. The person should avoid overstimulating, emotionally charged, or conflict situations such as violent movies, newspapers, work issues, family conflicts or stressful demands for two hours before bedtime. Exercise should not be done during this time, as Yoga, Tai Chi or aerobic activity can energize the body so that sleep is difficult. Exercise should be scheduled into the early part of the day or in the early evening before supper. There should be no eating or drinking (except water) after 7 or 8 PM. The last two hours of waking time should be allocated for pleasant, relaxing activities. The bedroom should be separate from household activities and should be dark, quiet, and a comfortable temperature.

Changing sleep habits is a lifestyle choice just as much as changing eating or exercise habits. The client may encounter resistance from family members who are used to having her available for homework, housework, cooking, and other family demands until late into the evening. These patterns should to be addressed within the family unit so that other household members can support the client with changing her sleep habits.

Acupressure points which can be used for promoting good sleep include: PC-6, HT-7, GB-20, GV-16, UB-38, GV-24.5 (brow chakra point), Ren-17, KI-6, UB-62   Table 12 summarizes acupoints which are useful in fibromyalgia and chronic fatigue syndrome.

SPECIALIZED TREATMENT TECHNIQUES

Moxibustion

Also known as "moxa" is a method used for heating individual acupoints or larger areas on the body. It is an extremely tonifying type of treatment and is useful for building up Qi, relieving cold, and warming the person. It can also be used to move stagnation in the channels, which leads to reduction in pain. Moxa is an herb called "mugwort" (Artemsia vulgaris), and is available in a number of different forms. Loose moxa is commonly used in China and Japan, but not so much in Western nations; small bits of the loose plant fiber are rolled into little balls, cones, or oblong shapes, placed directly on the acupoint, and ignited. This type of treatment is called "direct moxa". Moxa is also available as cigar-sized rolls which are lit, and the burning end is held over the area to be treated so that the radiant heat enters the point or larger area. This is called "indirect moxa". It is also available in compact sticks like incense which fit into a ball-point pen sized instrument called a "tiger-warmer", and the acupoints are warmed with this. Other types are available as well, including smokeless moxa rolls and stick-on moxa.

Indirect moxa is very simple to use. The main precaution is to avoid overheating the point. Ask the client to verbally indicate when she can feel the heat The practitioner should frequently touch the area being warmed to detect the heat. The skin should be slightly pink when the appropriate amount of heat has been applied. Most clients enjoy moxa, and become deeply relaxed and warm after the treatment.

Magnets

Tiny bio-magnets are available which can be used to treat individual points. Since the human being generates an electromagnetic field, magnets can be used to manipulate the field. Qi may be the same thing as the electromagnetic field, and stagnation and deficiency of Qi may correspond to aberrations in the field. The Qi moves from magnetic north to magnetic south, so when a north pole magnet is placed next to the skin, it disperses Qi in that area; when the south pole is placed next to the skin, it attracts Qi to that area.

North pole magnets are placed over areas where pain occurs, as pain, by definition, is a stagnation pattern. A south pole magnet may be placed on an acupoint of the same energetic channel further downstream to draw Qi in its natural healthy direction. Magnet therapy is extremely powerful, and as with all techniques discussed, should not be attempted without proper instruction and thorough knowledge of the polarity of the magnets and the location of treatment points.

Some clients find that other types of magnetic products such as wrist bands, shoe insoles, or back braces containing magnets are helpful for relieving pain and discomfort. These are available from oriental medical supply vendors.

Cupping

Cupping is an ancient Chinese used to treat areas of stagnation. It is commonly applied along the muscles of the back and the large joints of the body such as the shoulders and hips. Glass or plastic cups are evacuated with the use of a flame or a suction pump and placed on the areas where localized blood stagnation, or ischemia, are found. The vacuum pulls the flesh up into the cup, and the result is often a slight to dramatic development of pink to purple color where the cups were placed. The more intense the color change, the more effective the procedure is in relieving stagnation.

The cups remain in place for two to ten minutes. Many clients report dramatic improvement of tightness, stiffness, or aching in the area within minutes of removing the cups. Frequently droplets of moisture appear on the skin inside the cup; excess fluids may actually be pulled out of the tissues by this method. The color fades away over a few days, and positive effects are quite long lasting. In many cases a few minutes of cupping can relieve stagnation better than several sessions of deep massage, is more comfortable for the client, and safer for the practitioner's hands. The procedure sometimes feels "weird" to the client, but if appropriate vacuum is used, it is not at all uncomfortable. Before using cupping, be sure the client is aware there may be temporary discoloration in the area being treated.

Chapter 6. Treatment Principles and Methods

TABLE 12.   ACUPOINTS FOR FIBROMYALGIA and CHRONIC FATIGUE SYNDROME

Point Number	Energetic Effect	Experiential Effect
Bladder-10	Removes channel obstructions, soothes sinews	Clears brain; helps memory; relieve neck & back tension & headache
Bladder-15	Invigorates Blood; calms the Shen; clears Heat	Helps anxiety and insomnia; calms the mind; helps depression
Bladder-17	Nourishes and invigorates Blood; releases diaphragm	Frees the breathing; calms the mind; soothes the stomach & digestion
Bladder-18	Resolves Damp Heat; moves stagnant Qi	Abdominal distension; depression; releases "wound up" feeling
Bladder-20	Tonifies SP & ST; resolves Dampness; nourishes Blood	Helps achiness; boosts energy; calms and balances digestion
Bladder-22	Regulates 3 Burners; resolves Lower Burner Dampness	Helps urinary problems, leg swelling and pain; edema
Bladder-23	Tonifies kidneys; nourishes blood; resolves Dampness	Energy boosting point; strengthens all body functions
Bladder-54 (40)	Removes obstructions in Bladder meridian	Relieves pain in legs and lower back
Du-4	Tonify Kidney Yang; expel Cold; strengthens the back	Energy booster; helps low back pain; warms the body
Du-14	Regulates Qi; Tonifies Yang; several meridians cross.	Clears the mind; stimulates brain; boosts energy; relieves fatigue
Gall Bladder-20	Eliminates Wind; subdues Liver Yang; clears brain	Relieves dizziness/ vertigo; neck & shoulder pain and headache
Gall Bladder-21	Remove channel obstructions; several meridians cross	Relaxes sinews; relieves neck and shoulder pain or stiffness
Gall Bladder-30	Clears channel obstructions; tonifies Qi and Blood	Energy booster; powerful whole-body balancing point
Gall Bladder-34	Gathering Pt for sinews; promote smooth flow of Liver Qi	Helps tendons, ligaments, muscles the body; anxiety & insomnia
Gall Bladder-40	Relieves stagnant Liver Qi; Source point of Gall Bladder	Helps depression, anxiety, irritability; decision making; stomach pain
Gall Bladder-41	Opens Dai Mai; resolves Damp Heat; smoothes Liver Qi	Migraines; irritability; depression; hip and knee Pain
Large Intestine-4	Harmonizes Qi ascending & descending	Boosts energy; relieves pain
Large Intestine-10	Tonifies Qi and Blood; clears LI channel	Boosts energy; helps arm pain
Large Intestine-11	Resolves Damp Heat; regulates Qi	Boosts energy; relieves achiness
Large Intestine-16	Moves channel blockage; regulates Qi	Benefits joints; opens the chest
Liver-3	Liver Source Pt ; promotes smooth flow of Liver Qi	Depression, anger; irritability; Liver detox function; stress relief

TABLE 12. ACUFOINTS FOR FIBROMYALGIA and CHRONIC FATIGUE SYNDROME

Point Number	Eneretic Effect	Experiential Effect
Liver-4	Promotes smooth flow of Liver Qi	Depression, anger; irritability; Liver detox function; stress relief
Liver-13	Gathering Point of Yin Organs	Supports building up of many types deficiency; builds Qi and Blood
Lung-5	Moves LU Qi down; clears phlegm	Boosts energy; reduces achiness
Lung-7	Circulates Defensive Qi; moves Qi Down	Settles achiness; supports immune
Lung-9	Regulates Lung Qi; clears Dampness	Boosts energy; reduces achiness
Namikoshi Extra	Removes channel blockages in hips and legs	Releases pain and stiffness in low back, hips, legs, sciatica
Pericardium-6	Regulates Qi and Blood; clears 3 burners; calms Shen	Powerful emotional stabilizer; used for anxiety, depression, and pain
Ren-4	Tonifies Kidneys and Original Qi	Energy boosting point
Ren-6	Tonifies Qi & Yang; regulates Qi; resolves Dampness	Use Moxa for extreme physical & mental exhaustion and depression
Ren-12	Resolves Damp; tonify digestion	Smoothes digestion, helps achiness
Ren-17	Tonify Qi of Heart and Lungs	Energy booster; helps palpitations & breathlessness
Spleen-3	Source Pt; strengthens Spleen; resolves Damp	Boosts energy; improves digestion; boosts energy
Spleen-4	Move Stagnation; Tonify SP/ST; relieves abdominal fullness	Improve digestion; relieve bloating; regulate menstruation
Spleen-6	Tonify Lower Burner; nourishes Blood & Yin	Helps digestion & menstruation; builds energy; helps achiness
Spleen-9	Resolves Damp; removes channel obstructions	Helps achiness and swelling, especially of legs, knees, feet
Spleen-10	Cools, moves, and tonifies the Blood	Used for painful or irregular menstrual periods
Spleen-21	Master Luo Point; moves blood in connecting channels	Used for generalized muscular pain throughout the body
Stomach-29	Relieves Blood Stagnation	Helps menstrual difficulties and pain
Stomach-30	Tonifies Pre- and Post- Heaven Qi	Energizes the body; helps digestion
Stomach-36	Tonifies Qi & Blood; expels Cold, wind, damp	Boosts energy; diminishes pain and achiness

Magraine (Ion) Pellets

Ion pellets are tiny (about 1 mm diameter) stainless steel spheres which can be purchased with gold or other types of metallic coating on them. Each pellet has its own adhesive plaster, and the pellets can be placed on specific treatment acupoints, or simply on tight, sore, or congested areas. They may be left in place as much as three to seven days, and the adhesive plasters seem to endure quite well for that length of time.

The pellets work in several useful ways. First, they provide a mechanical stimulation to the point, similar to the effects of massaging the point. Secondly, since gold is an excellent conductor of electricity, gold pellets placed on points of the same energetic pathway actually facilitate the flow of Qi along the pathway, thus relieving stagnation and the pain and discomfort which accompanies it. Thirdly, they can serve as landmarks for points which the client is asked to massage as homework.

The pellets are discarded after use, and the client only needs to be made aware of their presence and purpose, and instructed to remove them if any local irritation occurs, or after a prescribed period of time given by the therapist. Use of ion pellets can extend the beneficial effects of the office visit for several days when appropriate treatment points are chosen.

Electro-acupuncture

Electro-acupuncture has been shown to be effective for the treatment of symptoms of fibromyalgia (Deluze et al, 1992). In this technique the needles are connected to each other with electrical wire, and an electronic device is used to transmit a weak current through the wires and needles to stimulate the points.

SUMMARY

All the techniques discussed here require sufficient knowledge and mastery of traditional Chinese medical theory and practice. They are powerful and effective, even though they may be perceived as unusual or strange to many Western clients. After they experience the positive effects, they will no longer be skeptical or suspicious. Use of these methods is as commonplace and accepted in Asian countries as aspirin or alka-seltzer is in the United States. It is important to educate clients so they understand the methods being used. It is in the best interest of both client and practitioner for these methods to be fully accepted and understood by the client at a non-technical level. They are all means of activating and releasing the body's own healing energies and abilities, and are therefore natural, non-invasive, and empowering therapeutic methods.

Chapter 7

Body-Mind Concepts for Pain Management

Pain is one of the most common symptoms which causes people to seek assistance from a health care professional. Physicians, massage therapists, acupuncturists, oriental bodywork therapists, chiropractors, and others have a high percentage of clients whose chief or secondary complaint is pain somewhere in the body. Of course, body pain is one of the cardinal symptoms of fibromyalgia. Working with clients who have chronic pain is interesting and challenging for the practitioner, and results tend to be much better when the practitioner works holistically.

In a study at the University of Maryland's Center for Complimentary Medicine, researchers identified back pain, arthritis and fibromyalgia as the chronic pain syndromes that contribute the greatest clinical and economic burden to overall chronic pain statistics. Not coincidentally people with these diagnoses are also users of alternative and complementary therapies. The Center has identified acupuncture, homeopathy, manual/ manipulative therapies, and mind-body therapies as the alternative medical therapies offering the greatest clinical potential for these three chronic pain diagnoses (Berman, 1997).

In this chapter we will explore a number of factors which contribute to the generation and perpetuation of pain. Many of the factors are mental and emotional, and this brings us into the realm of the holistic paradigm. Other factors have to do with simple lifestyle modification and other choices; the practitioner who serves as a partner, facilitator, and educator for her/his clients can offer many suggestions that clients can do for themselves at home. By providing concepts in this chapter, rather than specific technique protocols, the practitioner can arrive at a greater understanding of the dynamics of pain. Understanding concepts at a deeper level will allow the practitioner to develop creative individualized techniques to work with each client's particular needs.

Teaching the client to care for herself is perhaps the highest form of health care. It empowers the individual to learn to know her body, emotional and mental states and environment in much more meaningful and powerful ways that relate to her health and comfort. It is one of the most rewarding outcomes for a practitioner to see a client who was dependent and needy transform into an empowered human being who has attitudes and skills to take care of her own health and well-being.

1. Physical Pain is a Universal Experience

At one time or another every person experiences pain of some kind. For most of us, our experience with pain starts at a very young age, with a bump on the head or knee, an upset stomach, or a sore throat. Most childhood pain is temporary unless there is an extreme trauma which sets the stage for long-term pain. The child in pain screams and cries until his caretakers come to his aid. The caretaker then begins to uncover the cause of the problem and administer a remedy. Many times the remedy is emotional comforting. If the adult caretaker cannot determine the cause of the problem or a solution for it, the child is usually taken to a medical practitioner.

We learn very early that when there is pain we need to seek external help. For children this is appropriate. Acute pain from injury or illness is an alarm to bring attention to the problem and potentially prevent more serious problems. However, when we grow up, we are much more likely to develop chronic pain. The accumulation of all the smaller shocks and traumas to the body finally catches up with many of us. Car accidents, sports injuries, falls, surgery, dental work, birthing, all add up over time. It is very rare to find an adult over age forty who does not have chronic pain somewhere in her/his body. Even teenagers can have fibromyalgia, headaches, and other types of chronic pain.

The practitioner needs to be aware of the ubiquitous nature of pain. For many people, even good therapy and self-care may only reduce pain rather than eliminate it. In many cases it will not be eliminated completely, and ironically, many of the clients have been going from practitioner to practitioner, mainstream and complementary, looking for a treatment which will totally eliminate their physical discomfort. The wise practitioner will assist the client in shifting to a point of view of looking for optimal relief and maximizing comfort and functionality. The more chronic the pain, the more difficult it is to resolve (see No. 5 below).

Many people with fibromyalgia can have totally pain-free periods of time which may last for a day, a week, or even months. However, the odds are very high that they will also have days which are not so good. The goal is to make the journey of life as comfortable and pleasant as we can while learning the lessons that pain, the great teacher, has to offer.

2. Pain is a Subjective Experience

It cannot be objectively measured. There is no blood test, radiograph, or computerized scan that can give a quantitative evaluation of a person's body sensations. The experience of pain is very personal in terms of quality and quantity. People vary in their pain thresholds. Many individuals learn to "tune out" their body awareness so they can get on with the activities of their lives. Others have more difficulty detaching and seem to be overwhelmed by their pain. Of course neither extreme is ideal; as a message pain may prevent us from causing further injury or damage to a painful area, and may motivate us to do something to remedy the situation. The best balance is to be able to "listen" to our bodies without becoming obsessed or overwhelmed with health challenges.

Numerous other factors influence the perception of pain.   Mental distractions and other demands may temporarily take one's mind off the pain. Sometimes people are surprised to find that when they get involved with something, pain such as a headache may disappear from awareness while they are occupied with other matters.

For practitioners working with clients who have chronic pain, it is important to create a pain map in the initial interview. In Chapter 5 it was recommended to have the client color a body chart indicating the areas of discomfort. The practitioner should also make a separate map indicating the areas of pressure pain, palpable tension, heat or cold, and structural imbalances such as scoliosis or leg-length discrepancies.

Calibration for pain is done subjectively. A scale of 1-10 works well. With the client lying comfortably on the treatment table, the therapist will carefully palpate, starting with the areas of pain the client has indicated on the chart they colored previously. It is often very helpful to identify and label which meridians are involved, and palpate other points on the involved meridians. For example, if the client complains of neck pain along the Urinary Bladder meridian, there will often be painful areas in the lumbar, sacrum, or calf muscles, all relating to the same meridian. This careful search may uncover distal points which will be useful in therapy. Many times the client was previously unaware of the tension outside the chief complaint area, and is surprised and favorably impressed when the therapist can easily locate other areas which are involved in the overall pattern.

Look for the pain pattern to occur in three dimensions. For shoulder and upper back pain, there are usually reactive points in the pectorals or sternum; for lumbar pain, carefully check the psoas and inguinal ligament areas in front for posterior neck pain, check the front of the throat and the sacrum and coccyx. Many times there will be other areas which need to be released to get lasting improvement. This is especially true for chronic pain.

3. Pain is in a Recursive Feedback Loop with "Stress"

Stress will frequently increase the perception of pain and pain may increase the stress responses of the body/mind, because pain is, in itself, another form of stress. Emotional and physical fatigue also increase the perception of pain. One of the pain management strategies the therapist can teach the client is to "listen" for oncoming fatigue, and take breaks from the activities before fatigue becomes extreme. Attention should be given to mental and emotional fatigue as well as physical fatigue.

4. The Subjective Experience of Pain is Related to the Individual's Perceptions of Time

In chronic pain situations the person has memory of all his past pain. Pain may be linked in a variety of ways to his memory of the past and can shade otherwise pleasant memories. Each day the chronic pain continues, he is increasing his memory bank of experiences in which pain was a factor.

People with chronic pain may also project their pain into the future. Expectation or fear of future pain can influence the decisions the person will make, and may cause him to be filled with dread of events or activities in which the pain may prevent him from participating, or of being dependent on others, or having to do necessary tasks such as going to work while enduring the pain.

The more the person stays in "present time", the time factor in chronic pain is reduced.   Milton H. Erickson, MD, was a hypnotherapist who did a great deal of work with individuals in chronic pain. He may have been the first to identify and utilize this concept in therapy with chronic pain clients. (Erickson, 1983).

Meditation is, among other things, training in keeping one's attention in present time. Qi Gong, Yoga, Tai Chi, and other kinds of deeply meditative movement or postures can be extremely beneficial for individuals learning to manage pain more effectively.   Kabat-Zinn (1990) describes meditative exercises taught to chronic pain clients at the Stress Reduction Clinic and the University of Massachusetts Medical Center.   The practitioner can teach simple movement and meditation techniques to interested clients.

5. Body Armoring and Compensatory Tension Patterns

Body armoring occurs in response to pain as a defense mechanism to protect an injured area.   Chronic pain often leads to chronic armoring patterns in the musculo-skeletal and visceral systems. The changes seem to occur in the energy field as well as in the physical tissues; skilled practitioners can detect them in the meridian flows and in the subtle energy bodies. Compensation patterns also develop as an adaptation to injury or pain. In order to remain upright and mobile in the gravitational field, muscle tension patterns change in the short run and in the long run.

Over time, armoring and compensation patterns become encoded into the "normal" postural and structural habitus of the individual. Observing the client's walking gait, sitting postures, and relaxed positioning on the treatment table can give important clues about these patterns.   Some readily observable ones to look for include head-forward posture, head tilts, one or both shoulders held high, rounded shoulders, concavity of the chest, shallow breathing, sway back, no lumbar curve, one hip higher, tight gluteals, tight adductors, hard belly, leg or foot turn-out, knock knees, foot drag, and leg length discrepancy.

Massage, bodywork, acupuncture, and other forms of physiotherapy can be used to release armoring patterns. New, more adaptive responses may be facilitated as well. Relaxation methods, meditation, visualization, and imagery are all viable options for chronic pain clients to use at home and work.   The therapist may act as an instructor to assist in the learning process. Systematic gentle movement such as Qi Gong, Yoga, Tai Chi, Sotai, or Feldenkrais exercises are very beneficial for re-educating the body to more adaptive postures and movement patterns. Therapeutic exercise such as these also incorporate correct breathing with the movements.

6. Neurological Pathways

The body does not seem to distinguish between physical sources of pain and emotional or mental sources of pain. It uses the same neurological pathways for both, and frequently they become neurologically coupled. Thus, many people notice that particular emotional responses or mental activities are highly correlated with physical pain. Anger may bring on a headache or shoulder tension; thinking about work tasks or problem solving may generate stiffness in the spine or hips.

7. Pain is the Result of Something NOT MOVING

According to traditional Chinese medicine, pain is always derived from some type of stagnation pattern. Stagnation of Blood or Qi can be caused by an underlying deficiency, or by the presence of a pernicious influence. Cold and Damp pathogens are common causes of stagnation and pain in the body.

From Western physiology's point of view we can identify additional substances or processes which, when blocked, create physical pain. Lymph, blood, neurological impulses, thoughts, digestive material, cerebrospinal fluid, joints, and muscles are all designed to move and flow. When any of these are not moving appropriately, the individual is likely to experience pain sooner or later.

From this simple concept of non-movement as a cause of pain, the therapeutic strategy becomes self-evident. Re-introducing movement into the area, substance, or process will bring a reduction in pain sensations. Keeping it moving over time leads to long term improvement. Therapists can use passive range-or-motion during hands-on sessions and recommend and instruct the client in stretching and light exercise at home.

If an area has been rigid and armored for a long period of time, movement can be painful at first. For clients with fibromyalgia body therapy and exercise are often uncomfortable in the beginning; proceed carefully and slowly. Staying in verbal communication with the person is important. It lets the therapist know how the person is feeling moment-to-moment, and allows the client to feel more in control of the situation.

Acupuncture, massage, shiatsu, tuina, Jin Shin Do, Jin Shin Jyutsu, Amma, passive stretching, and many other modalities and approaches will get the Qi and Blood moving. When pain is chronic, ongoing movement practices will be necessary to maintain the benefits of therapy. The client must learn to participate in therapeutic activities, as listed above, at home to achieve lasting improvement. If they stop moving, pain will usually return within days.

8.   Generalization and Deletion Patterns of Thinking

Two common mental patterns influence the client's perception of pain in his/her body. Some people have a tendency to generalize pain to "everywhere, all the time". Frequently, generalization is a theme in their lives, and they tend to universalize many things. They will use universal quantifier words like "always, never, everywhere, no where, everybody, nobody, totally, completely, nothing, everything", and so on. This type of person is quite susceptible to feeling overwhelm, fear and hopelessness in life, because this pattern of thinking places things in discrete boxes without mechanisms to move in, out, or among the boxes. Their pain or other symptoms can easily become the centerpiece of their life and they can tend toward obsessive thinking.

For this type of client it is important to teach body awareness. Bodywork and exercises are excellent methods for learning to make distinctions in body sensations. Body scan meditation or progressive muscle relaxation exercises which can be done at home, and body mapping in the clinical session can be excellent methods. It is also beneficial to help the person identify exceptions to her universalizing. For example, to a statement like "Nobody understands anything that I'm going through", the therapist could ask the client to think of just one person who might have an inkling of understanding.

Other people with chronic pain learn to "tune it out", thus decreasing their body awareness and communication with their body. They tend to think in terms of deletions much of the time, deleting portions of their experience which do not fit into their model of the world, or which induce powerful negative emotions such as fear or anger. Sometimes this is called "denial", and it can occur consciously or unconsciously.

This type of person frequently feels a sense of anger at his own body or feels betrayed by his body. Individuals who have over-identified with their physical body, it terms of athletic ability, physical beauty, or sexuality can easily fall into this trap of denial. The very body which was once their source of self esteem and power over others has failed them, so they disassociate from it. Many times this type of individual feels his symptoms and illness are out of control like a mutinous crew. The body, formerly a source of pride and self-esteem, may become the enemy, preventing the person from doing what he wants to do.

This type of individual may have a difficult time giving information to the therapist. He may have a hard time describing the location or quality of body sensations, may exhibit a high degree of armoring, may under-report symptoms, and may regard physical illness or symptoms as weakness of character. He may also tend to expect dramatic, instantaneous change from the therapy; this type person is more likely to drop out of therapy before getting benefits if he does not see rapid progress.

9. Secondary Gain

Chronic illness, disability, and pain all have the potential to create opportunities for secondary gain. This means that some benefit is derived from the condition. The individual may be conscious or unconscious of these patterns which develop over time. Secondary gain can come in many forms, from dependency on financial support because of the disability, to attention, sympathy, or manipulation of friends and family members based on the illness or pain.

The deeper cause of secondary gain is usually conflict, either internal or external, or unmet needs. Examples could include the needs of self versus needs of others, job versus family, cultural expectations versus personal expectations, or childhood programming versus reality by experience.

When secondary gain exists, it can become an important perpetuating factor in the illness or pain. Usually these deeper conflicts occur at the unconscious level, and the individual may first need to become aware of them before they can change. If the practitioner is not trained to work with these situations, it is best to refer the client to a counsellor or support group which can help uncover and resolve these conflicts. Twelve-step programs are excellent formats for this type of work, and self-help books can be beneficial for the person who enjoys reading and is motivated to do inner work.

Below are four questions to assist with the soul-searching required to uncover secondary gain from pain or illness. Each could be the topic of discussion in a therapy session, or the subject of journaling, or an object for meditative reflection.

- What would happen if I continue to have this pain (illness)?
- What would happen if I didn't have this pain (illness)?
- What wouldn't happen if I continue to have this pain (illness)?
- What wouldn't happen if I didn't have this pain (illness)?

10. Pain as Communication

Clients frequently regard pain as an annoyance, a problem, a distraction, something to be eliminated, but they rarely regard it as a message or signal from the body. It is an important shift in awareness when the client can begin to regard his pain as communication. Information may be about the source or cause of a problem, or about which things make it better or worse. Pain can tell the person much about the stressors in his life, and the person who can develop the ability to "read" his pain signals will develop a different relationship with his body.

In it's earliest role as a messenger, pain is an adaptive response by the body to get the person's mental attention. If the message is ignored or handled inappropriately, often the body will escalate its attempt to get attention. The pain may increase in duration, intensity, location, or quality. At this point the body is making a request for some kind of intervention. If this request is ignored, the next stage will be a demand. More increase in intensity, locations, or duration of pain may ensue. Finally, the message of "do or die" is sent. Pain may become so intense it cannot be ignored, or other symptoms such as bleeding or loss of consciousness may occur.

11. Locus of control (Who's in Charge?)

Locus of control refers to the allocation of power and control in the client's life. Quite frequently, individuals who are disabled by their pain and other symptoms have their locus of control outside themselves. They may give their personal power to their mate, other relatives, physician, or even to their insurance provider.

A study of post-polio syndrome patients, which exhibit symptoms remarkably similar to fibromyalgia, identified several relevant correlations (Kuehn et al, 1994). Subjects with chronic diseases more often demonstrated external locus of control in contrast to people taking preventive health actions, who tended to believe more in internal or personal control over health status. Subjects with an internal locus of control orientation are able to cope more adaptively in response to stressful situations and are less vulnerable to the effects of chance and powerful others than are those subjects with external control beliefs. Subjects with a higher internal health locus of control score identified more coping resources than those whose locus of control was with powerful others.

Researchers found that symptom distress decreased as coping resources increased. Occurrence of symptom distress and the extent of severity of the symptom distress were both significantly negatively correlated with coping resources. Coping resources are identified as cognitive, social, emotional, spiritual/philosophical, and physical.   Examples could include problem solving skills (cognitive), support from family and friends (social), journaling or counselling (emotional), faith in a higher power (spiritual), and exercise or stretching (physical). All these methods can be incorporated into an effective stress management program.

Cognizance of a client's locus of control can create more individualized plans for client's coping styles, sick-role definition, learning patterns, problem-solving, preventive techniques, and adaptive techniques. See also the section on Self-Efficacy in Chapter 3.

The shift of locus of control from external to internal represents a significant transformational process. Some of the elements which may need to be addressed by an individual to make this transformation may include:

- Overcoming victim thinking
- Dealing with self esteem issues
- Reclaiming authority from "Powerful Others"
- Learning appropriate boundaries

12. Oxygen Deprivation Increases Pain and Fatigue

Oxygen is necessary for the tissues and organs to function normally. Oxygenating the system reduces pain and fatigue. There are many techniques which can be used in the clinic or at home which will improve the oxygenation of the body. Refer also to Chapter 8 (Rebuilding the Immune System) for more information about these topics. The following list gives a number of methods for improving oxygenation.

- Consciously working with breathing to develop abdominal (Hara) breathing. This can bring more air into lungs and improves the exhalation phase. This makes more oxygen available for absorption and facilitates removal of waste products through the lungs.
- Movement (distributes oxygen to tissues via blood flow).
- Environmental considerations (pollutants may compete with oxygen).

- Physiological problems such as anemia, asthma, emphysema, circulation problems, and diabetes affect the body's ability to absorb or transport oxygen.
- Supplements such as green drinks, anti-oxidants, miso and proper nutrition support the body's ability to absorb, transport and utilize oxygen.
- Bodywork for diaphragm, spine, ribs, and muscles of respiration can release armoring that inhibits proper breathing and increase the client's awareness of his breathing patterns.
- Stretches and exercise for the diaphragm, spine, ribs and muscles of respiration contribute to release of armor.
- Specific breathing exercises can help the individual retrain and develop awareness of proper breathing.
- Aerobic exercise improves cardiovascular fitness, making heart and lung functioning more efficient.

13. Common Fears and Illusions Regarding Pain

Fear is an emotion which suspends motion and stops activity. It causes Qi to become stagnant and rigid, especially in the Kidneys and Heart. Underneath each fear is an illusion that feeds the fear and keeps it alive. Many times individuals are not even consciously aware of the depth and intensity of their fears, and of how much their fears govern their lives. Fears erode self esteem and confidence, undermine hope, shatter positive expectations, and steer a person's decisions. The thoughts and feelings we maintain in our minds and bodies radiate particular qualities of energy. Actions and decisions which are fear-based are eventually doomed to failure because the "Law of Attraction" magnetically draws to us exactly what we fear most. Those are the types of experiences which resonate with our internally generated mental and emotional states.

The therapist can help the client bring his fears into conscious awareness by thoughtful conversation exploring the issues which influence that person's life. Once the fears are identified, the person can begin to uncover the illusions which drive them and keep him stuck in illness and pain. In many cases, awareness is the key to finding an antidote to the fears and illusions. Table 13 is a list of common fears and illusions among people who have chronic pain or illness, including fibromyalgia and chronic fatigue. The four questions at the end of Section 11 on secondary gain may also be used to help uncover fears and illusions.

Table 13. Common Fears and Illusions About Pain and Illness

> - Fear of always having pain
> - Fear of worsening pain
> - Fear of giving up medications such as pain pills or other "crutches"
> - Fear of something "really wrong" but undetected, such as tumors or MS
> - Fear of the unknown
> - Fear of change
> - Fear of relaxing, feeling of "coming apart" or losing control when body armor releases
> - Illusion of pain as "punishment" for wrongful thoughts or deeds or for being a "bad person"
> - Illusion of matter more powerful than energy
> - Illusion of medical research "finding a cure" ; this places locus of control outside the individual and de-activates motivation to explore new methods and self-help techniques
> - Illusion of pain as a solitary experience
> - Illusion of doctor, medications, practitioner, or techniques "curing" illness
> - Illusion of being totally and permanently free of symptoms
> - Illusion of past situations or acts of other people as cause of pain or illness
> - Illusion of pain as only a physical problem- denial of stress and mental or emotional factors
> - Illusion that a doctor or health care practitioner knows more about them than they do; lack of trust in one's own experience and intuition

14. The Language of Pain

Linguistically, the word "pain" is a nominalization. Nominalizations are nouns which are derived from verbs, and represent a process frozen in time. Other familiar nominalizations include "relationship" (frozen form of relating), "communication" (frozen form of communicating), and "organization" (frozen form of organizing). The names of emotions are also nominalizations; anger, grief, fear, and joy are actually processes rather than fixed "things."

When we speak of "pain" we are making a process into a thing. A process is in dynamic fluctuation and susceptible to many influences, while a "thing" seems much more tangible and permanent. When speaking to clients, practitioners can shift their language to speak in process words more than nouns. This will allow the client's neurology to shift in ways that give them more internal resources for changing their symptoms. Example: Instead of saying "show me where the pain is," say "show me where you would like to feel better and move more easily."

Another linguistic strategy is to use less emotionally charged words. The word "pain" is emotionally charged, linked to the person's memories of past pain, his fears about the future, his emotional wounds, and much more.

Table 14 shows a series of words in decreasing intensity that can be used to take the emotional charge off the process. As the conversation progresses as part of the therapeutic process, the practitioner can use more of the less emotionally charged words.

Table 14. The Language of Pain

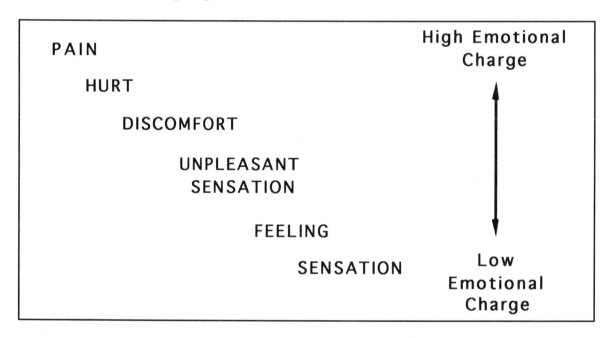

15. Distraction and Dilution as Therapeutic Strategies

Pain calls one's attention and awareness to the painful area; this makes pain a compelling messenger from the body. Other matters which command one's attention can draw attention away from the pain. Everyone has had the experience of being absorbed in an interesting activity and having a headache or toothache "disappear" while the attention is diverted.

In acutherapy or massage sessions there are times when techniques may be uncomfortable or painful. It is desirable to work within the client's range of perception of "no pain" up to and including "good hurt" sensations. When working with fibromyalgia clients the tissues can be so sensitive that even light touch elicits a painful response. Even light acupressure or meridian work may feel intense to these clients. When it is necessary to work painful points or meridians, the practitioner can use distraction techniques to divide the client's attention, reducing the perception of pain.

Verbal interaction is one way to accomplish this. Directing the client's attention verbally, or engaging her in observation of her body sensations can be very effective. Therapists who have training in hypnotherapy, neuro-linguistic programming, gestalt therapy, or other communication therapies can use metaphor, representation system overlap, guided imagery, and many other linguistic methods to shift the client's attention when necessary to deeper, more uncomfortable techniques during a bodywork session.

Creating more than one physical point of attention is also effective for diluting perceptions of discomfort. Most people cannot pay attention to more than two or three areas of their body simultaneously. With needling or hands-on therapy, it is usually possible to distract the client's attention from a painful area by simultaneously stimulating additional points or regions. For example, when working a painful Spleen-6 point, the therapist could simultaneously work Large Intestine-4, Liver-13, or another sensitive point.

16. Tracking Pain Variables to Monitor Progress in Therapy

Pain syndromes always has at least two variables that can be monitored for progress in therapy. The pain has an intensity, usually evaluated subjectively on a ten-point scale, and a quality. Qualities are descriptions such as sharp, stabbing, dull, aching, radiating, squeezing, throbbing, and so on. Pain which is present continuously, as in many cases of neck or low back pain, can be monitored over time. The client can keep track, giving each day a score, and noting activities or situations which cause the pain to worsen or improve. If the therapy is going well, the intensity will be going down over a period of time, and the quality will be changing to something more easy to live with. Table 15 shows a sample graph of pain intensity decreasing over time as therapy progresses.

Table 15. Changes in Pain Intensity Before and After Therapy

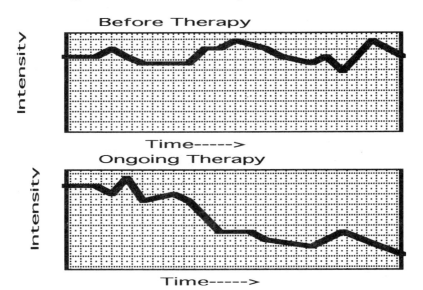

Pain which occurs intermittently, such as migraine headaches, menstrual cramps, or irritable bowel flare-ups, have two additional characteristics: duration of the pain episode, and the interval between episodes. Some people have migraines which last a week or longer; reducing the duration to one or two days would represent a vast improvement in their condition. Some people have migraines four times per month; reducing this to once per month would again represent an improvement, even if the intensity and duration remain the same. When working with episodic pain conditions, it would be most desirable to see improvement in all these variables, as diagrammed in Table 16.

Tracking changes in these variables over time illustrates that there are many ways to experience improvement in pain symptoms. It is also a method for getting clients more involved in their therapy, and for increasing their awareness of their patterns.

Table 16. Changes in Intensity, Duration, and Interval for Episodic Pain

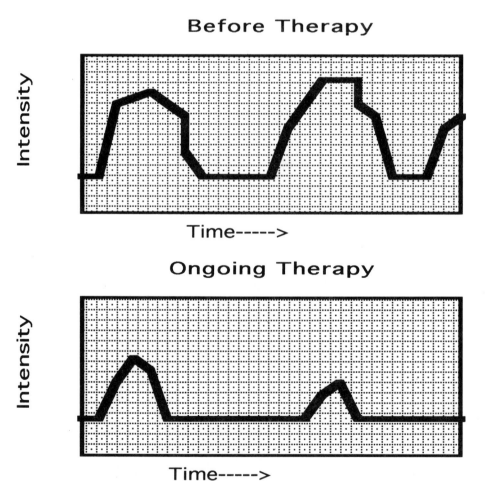

17. Make Realistic Therapeutic Goals

It is important to help the client set realistic goals for therapy. Getting the client involved in self-therapy and lifestyle changes will support progress. The practitioner can help the client explore options and assist with resources as needed. The practitioner should resist dictating or mandating what the client should do. The holistic paradigm emphasizes the partnership of client and therapist, with the client as the head of the team. In the beginning homework must be simple and well within the client's abilities and interests to generate experiences of success and self-empowerment.

The goal is NOT to achieve total disappearance of pain, but rather to work toward improvement of overall comfort and functionality. Focus on changing the qualities of pain and lowering the intensity. Have the client describe the qualities such as dull, heavy, draggy, sharp, cutting, twisting, burning, nagging, stabbing, biting, hot, cold, grinding, throbbing, gnawing pains. Map carefully, and review and update maps every four to six sessions.

Chapter 8

Rebuilding the Immune System

THE IMMUNE SYSTEM AND ILLNESS

Research suggests that individuals who have chronic fatigue syndrome have immune dysfunction (Gupta, 1991). Rebuilding the immune system is a vital part of recovering from a chronic illness. According to Elson Haas MD (1992), "Our immune system is the most dynamic body component in determining our state of health or disease." From the holistic point of view, the immune system is more than just the body's defense mechanism. It is the mechanism which allows the body-mind to identify "self" from "not-self". Thus, it is the physiological component of self identity. When the physiological immune system is faltering, it is analogous to the breakdown of one's personal integrity, identity, self-esteem. The breakdown of the immune system corresponds to the breakdown of the self. (See Signals of immune system suppression in Chapter 1)

Chinese medicine has a rich and complex understanding of what we know as the immune system. There are four types of immune deficiency relating to the Vital Substances. Blood deficiency type would involve anemia, blood toxicity, chronic acid blood, and poor circulation. Qi deficiency type is characterized by chronic fatigue, depression, dislike of movement and activity, loss of libido, and mental fatigue. Yin deficiency type appears as lymphatic impairment, poor tissue healing and repair, and lack of fluids in the body leading to false heat and symptoms of dryness such as dry eyes, dry skin, or lack of vaginal secretions. Yang deficiency type leads to weakened resistance to colds and flu, feeling cold or chilly frequently, exhaustion and chronic fatigue. Combinations are possible.

Three of the Organ/meridian systems have significant relationships to the immune system. The Lungs rule the Wei Qi, or defensive Qi, which is the closest concept that corresponds to the immune system of Western medicine. The Lungs provide the avenue for taking in air, extracting the Air Qi, and then discharging the unused portions of the air. Thus the Lungs are the interface between the individual and the environment in which he lives and exchanges matter and energy. The skin is the body tissue corresponding to the Lungs and the Metal element, and forms a boundary or interface between what is inside the person and what is outside. Symbolically, the Metal element serves as a shield or protective armor which defends and protects the individual from attack by harmful external forces. Metaphorically, then, the weakening or breakdown of this energetic field corresponds to the breakdown of the person's fundamental integrity as an individual in his own right. Unresolved grief or sadness injures the Lungs and Wei Qi. With a weakened Metal element and Lungs, the system has difficulty keeping "me" and "not me" separated.

The second Organ/meridian which has powerful influence on the immune system is the Spleen. The Spleen is in charge of the lymphatic system (see Chapter 9), which is an integral part of the immune system. The Spleen (sometimes called Spleen-Pancreas to acknowledge the coupled effects of these two Organs) is assigned to the Earth element in the Five Element system. Earth is the centering and grounding force; the substrate in which our energetic roots connect with the planetary energy. The Spleen, along with its partner the Stomach, is in charge of extracting the essence of ingested food, and is the starting place for the generation of Qi and Blood in the body. This is the second way we take in and internalize matter and energy from our environment. The Spleen and Lungs are in charge of the alchemical processes which turn "not me" into "me". When these functions are impaired the body will be limited in it's vitality. Poor quality diet, along with excessive thinking or worry injure the Spleen. Deficiency of the Spleen Qi is always a central imbalance in chronic fatigue and fibromyalgia.

The third meridian to consider when working with the immune system is the Triple Burner. The Triple Burner does not have an Organ as such, but is an integrative functional aspect of the body's energetic system. It has been described as regulating the fluid metabolism and distribution, as well as being closely associated with balance among the endocrine glands. It also correlates with functioning of the sympathetic nervous system, the "fight or flight" mechanism. The paired meridian is the Pericardium or Heart Governor, which correlates with the parasympathetic nervous system. The Triple Burner connects the eight extraordinary vessels and the source energy, or Yuan Qi, sometimes called the "moving Qi between the Kidneys," with the source points of all the meridians. Several of the endocrine glands, especially the adrenals, thymus, and thyroid, have roles in immune function according to Western physiology, so an integrative force among them gives us a powerful tool to use therapeutically.

The Triple Burner is the commander of the system, and it can move energetic resources to meet the ongoing needs of the person. It can override other body needs to ignite fever, release adrenaline, direct antibodies, and other activities to handle emergencies. An overactive Triple Burner, or one which is not adept at distinguishing "real" emergencies from false alarms, can set the stage for the development of illness, particularly chronic fatigue syndrome and auto-immune disorders. In these situations, the Triple Burner excess keeps the body's systems mobilized and in attack mode continuously.

Stress is closely connected to Triple Burner imbalance. Stress is, by some definitions, the body's response to challenges which may come from internal or external sources. In modern society, people often have high levels of stress coming from many sources (see Chapter 1). This keeps the Triple Burner chronically over-stimulated. Continuous negative emotions such as anger, worry, and fear are destructive to the immune system. Happiness, contentment, will power, patience, compassion, and confidence are mental/emotional states which strengthen the immune system.

Many aspects of lifestyle influence the functioning of the immune system. Some factors promote the immune system, while others contribute to its deterioration. In this chapter we will look at several of those factors.

REBUILDING THE IMMUNE SYSTEM

Sleep and Rest

Many people in our modern fast-paced culture are simply sleep-deprived. Sleep is a necessary process for healing, tissue repair, and stress release through dreams. Energetically, it is the Yin complement to the active Yang waking part of the day. Without appropriate amounts of sleep, the Yin energies of the body eventually become depleted. Yang arises out of Yin, so over time the person can become deficient in both.

For individuals with chronic fatigue or fibromyalgia, this is an excellent place to start rebuilding. It is important to set regular bedtime, regular time of arising, and have adequate hours allocated for rest and regeneration. Most people need seven to eight hours of sleep nightly to maintain health of the immune system. Those who are recovering from chronic illness may need more than this. Rest times during the day are also indicated. Individuals with these disharmonies usually crave more rest and sleep, but frequently feel driven by the demands of their job, family, or other responsibilities. They feel as if they are on a rapidly moving treadmill which is out of control, and to jump off would cause more damage than to continue the ceaseless over-doing lifestyle. If the pattern is not changed, the condition will only worsen over time.

When recovering from chronic illness, activities during the day must be metered in such a way as to conserve energy. The wise individual must learn her/his own limitations and be willing to honor them. Part of the pattern in the development of chronic fatigue and fibromyalgia is one of over-doing and running on empty (See the energy management strategy in Chapter 12).

In some lineages of Tai Chi and Qi Gong, students are taught the "seventy percent rule". In this approach, the student is instructed to confine his efforts to approximately seventy percent of his actual capacity. For example, if the student could practice two hours of Tai Chi, he should stop after one-and-one-half hours. If he could stretch a certain amount, he should only stretch seventy percent of that amount. All exertions are metered in this manner. Then the individual always has thirty percent of his energy in reserve for emergencies and unplanned demands which may occur from time to time. Tai Chi and Qi Gong are metaphors for life, teaching balance, moderation and development of self-mastery. Seventy percent is the recommendation for a balanced lifestyle for a healthy person. When someone is attempting to recover from illness, they should exert perhaps only forty to fifty percent of their full capacity, allowing half their time and energy for rest and regeneration. Healing requires a large expenditure of energy. This approach is markedly different from the typical Western approach which seeks to push patients to the limit when they are rehabilitating. The seventy percent rule is an excellent stress management guideline, and doing less than this when healing is perhaps a more "middle path" approach.

Application of the seventy percent rule in everyday life can be quite challenging for those who are used to a lifestyle of perpetually over-doing, but once a person becomes used to it and notices how much more relaxed h e feels, and how much more stress-hardy he is, he will be very reluctant to resume a lifestyle of extremes. One can apply this in most, if not all, activities, including career, house and yard work, reading or studying, social activities and time away from the home for errands and other tasks. It requires the individual to plan and organize better, delegate tasks to others, and prioritize to eliminate unnecessary or redundant activities. Reducing overall consumption of food and personal possessions would also be in line with this philosophy. A commitment to the seventy percent rule will result in simplifying one's life and always having an energy reserve.

Nutrition

Poor diet weakens the Spleen, creating deficiencies of Qi and Blood throughout the body. To rebuild the immune system it is essential to shift to a natural whole-foods diet. Whole grains and vegetables should form the bulk of the diet. Simple foods and simple meals are easier to digest and promote restoration of the immune system and other body systems. Use good quality sea salt instead of chemically manufactured salt which is sold in grocery stores. If digestion is sluggish or inefficient, do not drink liquids with meals, as this dilutes the digestive enzymes and over-fills the stomach and intestines.

Meat in small quantities is appropriate for most people; use organic poultry or fresh fish two or three times per week if meat is desired. Avoid beef and pork. Do not eat late at night or while working or studying. Eat meals i n pleasant surroundings with people who are supportive and caring. Do not discuss business, health problems, or stressful topics at meal times. Make meals a time of relaxation, centering and healing.

Addition of sea vegetables in cooking is a health-promoting choice. They add high quality minerals, fiber, and energetic support to the Organs, especially the Kidneys. Green drinks such as wheatgrass juice are also beneficial to the immune system. Wheatgrass juice is recommended for people with chronic fatigue. Most juice bars have fresh juice daily. Blue-green algae or tablets of barley greens are also valuable for boosting the immune system. Consider this if green drinks are not a suitable option. Those who have had much antibiotic therapy are also recommended to use acidophillus to replace intestinal flora. Many chronic fatigue sufferers have taken many antibiotics over the years. Restoring colon health can take weeks or months. Harmful foods and substances to avoid include the following:
- White sugar and flour
- Carbonated beverages and soft drinks
- Artificial sweeteners
- Fried foods
- Hydrogenated vegetable oils and margarine
- Dairy products (except butter)
- Chemical additives such as monosodium glutamate (MSG), preservatives, colorings, flavor enhancers
- Antibiotics and many other medications
- Alcoholic beverages
- Recreational drugs
- Tobacco

Nutritional Supplements for Immune Boosting

1. <u>Zinc</u> -- One of the most powerful immune system nutrients. Zinc improves T and B cell functioning, promotes thymic hormones, improves resistance to infection, and speeds tissue healing. Zinc has been identified as a co-factor in approximately seventy enzyme systems. Take 45-60 mg/day; the citrate form is easier to absorb. Zinc lozenges are readily available and are a good way to supplement zinc.

2. <u>Iron</u> -- Promotes cellular immunity and neutrophil activity.

3. <u>Selenium</u> -- Increases antibody response and reduces carcinogenesis of the cells; counteracts depression.

4. <u>Copper</u> -- Improves resistance to infection (3 mg./day).

5. <u>Folic Acid</u> -- Improves production of blood cells (800 mcg/day).

6. <u>Vitamin A</u> -- Promotes cellular immunity, promotes tissue healing, decreases susceptibility to infections, and improves immunoglobin levels. (10,000 units/day).

7. <u>Vitamin C</u> -- Improves wound healing, increases phagocytic activity, improves cellular protection, anti-oxidant. (4000 to 10000 mg per day, as much as can be tolerated without diarrhea).

8. <u>Vitamin E</u> -- Increases antibody responses and production, improves cell membrane integrity, anti-oxidant (400-800 units/day).

9. <u>Vitamin B complex</u> -- Lowers stress response, improves humoral and cellular immunity, increase metabolism, (take a balanced formula).

Acid-Alkaline Balance

An important but frequently overlooked aspect of using foods for healing is the acid-alkaline balance of the blood. Acidity and alkalinity is measured by units called pH; pH in nature can range from 1 to 14. pH 7 is neutral; below pH 7 is acidic, above pH 7 is alkaline. The pH of human blood plasma must remain at a constant level in the range of 7.35 to 7.45, which is just slightly to the alkaline side. If it falls as low as 6.95, which is slightly acid, the result is diabetic coma and death, and if it rises to 7.7, the result is tetanic convulsions and death. Diagram 4 shows a scale of pH values for common familiar substances.

Diagram 4. pH Values for Common Substances

ACID		NEUTRAL				ALKALINE
Stomach Acid (HCl)	Wine	Water	Blood	Sea Water	Baking Soda	
pH 1	pH 3.5	pH 7	pH 7.35 - 7.45	pH 8.1	pH12	

Blood pH below 7.35 is considered acid blood. Blood pH can be measured in a blood test administered by a physician, but with a little awareness and experience, most people can learn to sense how their blood pH is doing by paying attention to how they feel. The cardinal sign of acid blood is FATIGUE, which is extremely common in people with chronic fatigue syndrome or fibromyalgia. Here is a list of the symptoms which may develop in an acid-blood condition.

- Feeling tired, exhaustion
- Slower heartbeat
- Spacey, dizzy feeling; ungrounded
- Chronic Infections- Candida, Herpes, sinus, kidney, etc.
- Arthritic conditions
- Rheumatic conditions
- Sticky-sour taste in mouth upon awakening in the morning
- Nervous imbalances- mental fogginess, twitches, "restless leg", insomnia
- Emotional imbalances-- anxiety, depression, mood swings, easily upset
- Demineralization signs and symptoms which can include:
- Soft teeth- many cavities
- Osteoporosis
- Broken, soft, cracked nails

It is possible to begin to change the quality of the blood within two weeks of correct eating. Many illnesses and disorders which are associated with "chemical imbalances" in the body will shift when proper blood pH is restored. Table 17 is a list of foods and activities which affect blood pH. Please note that some foods which are acidic themselves have an alkalizing effect on the body. Citrus fruits are an example.

It is possible to change the quality of the blood within 2wks

Table 17. Foods and Activities Which Affect Blood pH

	Acid-Forming	Alkaline-Forming
Most Extreme Effect	Chemicals (preservatives, coloring)	Salt
	Drugs and medications	Miso- tamari
	Artificial sweeteners	Soy beans- lima beans
	Ice cream	Sea vegetables
	Fats and oils	Potatoes
	Sugar-refined white or brown	Green beans
	Red meat	Green peas
	Poultry and fish	Vegetables
	Eggs-cheeses-tofu-butter-milk	Whole fruits
	Honey and other sweeteners	Fruit juices
	Alcohol- tobacco	Coffee
	White flour	
	Legumes, white, red or brown	
Slight Effect	Unrefined flour	
	Whole grains	
Activities with Acid or Alkaline Effect	Muscular activity (lactic acid)	Deep breathing
	Muscular inactivity	Thorough chewing of food
	Stress	Sunlight exposure

Herbs

Herbal therapy can be valuable for rebuilding the immune system and recovering from fibromyalgia and chronic fatigue. Chinese herbs are used in formulations which usually consist of six to twelve single herbal ingredients. Many formulas are hundreds of years old, and well tested in clinical practice. Multi-herb formulations effectively remove the vast majority of potential undesirable effects, as no ingredient makes up more than fifteen or twenty percent of a formula. Complementary ingredients give balance and effectiveness. There are also several Western herbs which are valuable for immune building. Some of the more common ones are listed below.

Western: Garlic, rosemary, echinacea, peppermint, cloves, golden seal, reishi mushroom, white willow, red clover, sheep sorrel, licorice root, burdock root, parsley, red clover, sarsaparilla root, ginger, cayenne

Chinese: Astragalus, Ginseng, Ligustrum, Codonopsis, Schizandra fruit, Ganoderma, Ginkgo, and Gotu Kola.

Emotional and Spiritual Healing

Moving out of victim thinking and into an empowered state is essential for rebuilding the immune system. Research has shown that self-efficacy benefits the immune system (Wiedenfeld, 1990) (See also Chapter 3). Chronic emotional stress degrades the immune system. Forgiving anyone or anything the person believes has harmed him is fundamental to the healing process. Gratitude and appreciation are also basic attitudes for promoting health and healing. Love of self and others energizes and strengthens the immune system and promotes antibody production. Positive thinking, including enthusiasm, kindness, will-power, generosity, and service are other mental/emotional states in which the immune system flourishes. Rossi (1986) gives an excellent discussion of the role of stress, emotional responses, and their relationship to the immune system, along with strategies for working with these. Chinese Five Element system is a rich model for understanding the correlation of mental/emotional processes with physiological ones; Table 18 summarizes the five element emotional qualities.

Table 18. Five Element Emotional Qualities

	Water	Wood	Fire	Earth	Metal
Organ/ Meridians	Kidney Urinary Bladder	Liver Gall Bladder	Heart Small Intestine Pericardium Triple Burner	Spleen Stomach	Lungs Large Intestine
Balanced emotional or mental states	Will power Resolve Self-esteem Creativity	Patience, ability to advance and retreat appropriately	Compassion Forgiveness Love, Joy Leadership Communication	Confidence Nurturing Supportive of others Grounded	Kindness, Contentment Flexibility
Unbalanced emotional or mental states	Fear, insecurity Low self esteem Weak will power	Anger, irritability, Frustration, rage Need to control	Bitterness, hatred, unforgiving	Worry, over-thinking, obsessive	Grief, sadness sorrow, can't let go, inflexible
Related physical imbalances	Back pain Urinary infection Fatigue	Hypertension Headaches PMS Fibrocystic	Cardiac problem Hypertension Digestive upset Insomnia	Blood sugar imbalances, stomach problems Fatigue	Asthma, weak immunity, lung diseases, colon problems

Sunlight

Regular exposure to full-spectrum sunlight brings many healthful benefits. The pituitary and pineal glands receive light energy through the retina and optic nerve. These two endocrine glands work together as the "control tower" for the whole endocrine system. Many of the human bio-rhythms, such as sleep, are regulated by light. Depression, sleep disturbances, and other problems can arise from insufficient exposure (less than one hour per day) to full spectrum light. Sunlight is alkalizing to the blood, which helps with many symptoms (See the section on acid/ alkaline balance in this chapter).

Over one hundred body functions have been identified as having daily rhythms. The pineal and it's hormone melatonin, has documented effects on reproductive functions, growth, body temperature, blood pressure, motor activity, sleep, tumor growth, mood, and the immune system.

Fibromyalgia and chronic fatigue clients should spend some time outdoors each day without sunglasses. The light enters the body primarily through the eyes, so it is counterproductive to wear sunglasses. This can also be a time to relax with nature, if there are suitable areas nearby, or to spend time in one's yard or patio. Many helpful exercise methods are done outdoors, such as walking, swimming, bicycling, hiking. For those who sunburn easily, use a good quality sunscreen to protect the skin.

For indoor use one can purchase full-spectrum light bulbs which can be placed in lamps or light fixtures at work and at home. Encourage clients to put them in the kitchen, reading area, office, and other areas where they spend significant amounts of time. They can be purchased in most lighting stores and health food stores.

Gradual and consistent exposure to sunlight yields many beneifts which are the same as a gradual and consistent program of exercise (Lieberman, 1991):

- Decreased resting heart rate
- Decreased blood pressure
- Decreased respiratory rate
- Decreased blood sugar
- Decreased lactic acid in the blood after exercise
- Increased energy, strength, and endurance
- Increased tolerance to stress
- Increased ability of the blood to absorb and carry oxygen

Aromatherapy

Aromatic blends with immune-boosting properties can be used in clinical sessions, or clients can use them at home on a daily basis. Essential oils are discussed in greater detail in Chapter 10.

Breathing

Most people breathe poorly, and their tissues, blood, and brains are under-oxygenated. Oxygen raises blood pH, allows muscles and organs to relax and function correctly, improves mood, promotes sleep, and clears the thinking. Symptoms of fibromyalgia and chronic fatigue improve when clients develop greater awareness and mastery of breathing.

Armoring responses from stress can cause tightening of the diaphragm, intercostal muscles, and scalene muscles of the neck, which are all muscles of respiration. Many people are unaware that they breathe poorly. After receiving bodywork they often comment how much easier it is to breathe, but when muscle tension returns, the breathing decreases again. Over time, bodywork and acupuncture can produce relaxation in the muscles so the person can maintain better breathing. However, this is an area where individuals can greatly benefit themselves by becoming aware of their breathing patterns and by doing exercises to relax the chest and retrain the breathing reflex. Tai Chi, Qi Gong, and Yoga incorporate breath awareness in the exercises. Breathing exercises can also be learned from books on the subject (Zi, 1986).

Meditation and Qi Gong

Qi gong meditative exercise activates the parasympathetic nervous system, sometimes called the "relaxation response". The sympathetic branch gives us the "fight or flight" response for reacting to real or perceived threats to our safety. When the parasympathetic branch is activated the adrenal glands, which secrete stress hormones such as adrenaline and cortisol, get to rest. The stress hormones suppress the immune system. The fight or flight stress response mechanism evolved to handle physiological needs for short periods of time when the individual's life is in danger. When the stress response is invoked, other body systems are put in "standby" mode until the crisis has been handled. Digestion, sleep, reproductive activities, and immune activities are put on hold, while heartbeat, blood pressure, respiration, and muscular tone increase. In modern society, however, stress has become a chronic factor for many people, and their adrenals are overworked. Qi gong is an excellent exercise method for those with chronic stress related symptoms such as digestive problems, sleep disorders, hypertension, and muscular armoring.

Meditation is one of the most effective methods for stress reduction, grounding, and spiritual development. Meditation leads to body-mind integration, expands awareness, and offers connection to the Spiritual realm. There are dozens of methods of meditation, which can be classified into three broad categories, each with a different effect on the individual (Lade, 1998). These are summarized in Table 19.

Table 19. Three Meditation Traditions

Meditation Type	Active Concentration on a Fixed Reference Point	Visualization or Guided Imagery	Non-focused Awareness
Method	One-pointed attention on a fixed object which may be internal of external	Generate a series of internal images which play out a drama or sequence	Detached observation of the mind; making the mind still
Examples	Internal: mantra, symbol, chakra, acupoint, image External: candle, crystal, I mage of guru, mandala	Microcosmic orbit; Catholic meditation on the sacred heart of Jesus Healing visualiztions	Mindfulness Quiet sitting Breathing meditations
Purpose	Transcendence of body and mind; identify and bond with non-physical world; connection to God, Divinity and the Spirit world	Create feelings of unconditional love, forgiveness, compassion; invoke healing processes, identification with humans	Enter a non-focused meditative state; expanded awareness of greater reality; release desire and attachment; surrender; connect to root of life
Energetic Center	Brow Chakra Upper Dan Tien Mental Body	Heart Chakra Middle Dan Tien Emotional Body (Astral)	Sacral Chakra Lower Dan Tien Physical Body (Etheric)
Cosmology	Connection to Heaven	Connection to Humans	Connection to Earth
Yin/Yang Polarity	Active process (Yang)	Active and Passive Awareness, balanced in Yin/Yang polarity	Passive Process (Yin)
Signal of Excess or incorrect, or wrong intent in meditative practice	Feelings of dissociation or detachment from one's own emotions, and from other people; headaches, neck pain, lowering body temperature	Aggravation of existing emotional imbalances, chest pain, breathing difficulty; attachment to person or guru becomes excessive	Self-importance, libido increased, irritability, lower body symptoms in joints or muscles; raising body temperature
Traditions and Cultures	Hindu; Ayurvedic (India)	Tantric, Taoist, Christian Mysticism, Tibetan (Europe, Tibet, China)	Zen, Taoist (Japan, China)

DHEA

Chronic illness appears likely to be associated with clear-cut adrenoandrogen deficiency or levels well below the mean of DHEA levels (Shealy, 1995, 1996). Both these articles are available on-line, and give a comprehensive report and literature review of the work on DHEA and chronic illness including cancer, AIDS, and diabetes.

DHEA supplementation may be indicated for clients with fibromyalgia and chronic fatigue. It is best to consult with a naturopath, chiropractor, or holistically-oriented physician before using supplements. It is recommended to use the lowest amount which gives beneficial results. Start with 25 mg per day, and have the person observe how they feel for a week. If no change, increase to 50 mg per day, and observe again for a week. Continue up to as much as 200 to 400 mg per day. Once the client is feeling better, they can implement natural methods to boost DHEA, including many of the areas discussed in this chapter. The person may be able to reduce to a low amount or eliminate supplementation once the adrenals are rejuvenated.

Because the body produces DHEA when healthy, it is desirable to encourage the body to produce its own supplies. Supplementation should be thought of as "jump starting." Long term usage, if chosen, should be kept at low levels, around 25 - 50 mg per day. Current recommendations for those with personal or family history of breast or ovarian cancer, or other hormonally mediated cancers, are to avoid DHEA supplements. These individuals should use other methods to boost DHEA and the immune system (See other methods in this chapter).

A Possible Vaccine Connection to FMS and CFIDS

Since vaccines were developed in the first decade of this century, the medical profession has been aware of the adverse effects of vaccines on the immune system. The DTP vaccine has been implicated in epidemics of paralytic polio since 1909, and other illness including joint pain and swelling, Guillian-Barre syndrome, and childhood diabetes (Neustaedter 1996). Some individuals have developed chronic fatigue or fibromyalgia within a short time after receiving hepatitis B vaccines and flu shots (Affleck 1999).

The National Vaccine Injury Compensation Program and the US Court of Federal Claims have accepted a causal relationship between rubella vaccine in the US and some chronic arthropathy with an onset between one and six weeks after vaccine administration (Weibel, 1996). Preliminary research indicates that the role of Rubella immunization in the etiology of chronic fatigue syndromes deserves further study (Allen, 1988).

At the time of this writing, conclusive evidence one about a connection between vaccines and FMS or CFIDS is not available in the medical literature. Even if immunization is a component in the onset of fibromyalgia or chronic fatigue for some individuals, many more people receive vaccinations without these unfortunate consequences. Other factors must also be present concurrently, and Chinese medicine recognizes that multiple factors are always involved in the development of illness. Practitioners are encouraged to continue to update themselves for information on this potential link, and to share information with clients so that they make informed decisions about vaccinations for themselves and family members.

Aspartame

Aspartame, the artificial sweetener in Nutrasweet and Equal has recently come under attack by consumer awareness groups, and has been implicated in numerous health challenges, in spite of FDA's continued support of the substance. Research is contradictory, and individual reports of problems with the substance are abundant. Many individuals have reported that consumption of aspartame worsens the symptoms of chronic fatigue and fibromyalgia. Aspartame may mimic symptoms or worsen many medical illnesses, including arthritis, multiple sclerosis, Parkinson's disease, lupus, multiple chemical sensitivity syndrome, diabetes. epilepsy, Alzheimer's disease, chronic fatigue syndrome, lymphoma, Lyme disease, attention deficit disorder, panic disorder, depression and other psychological disorders. An on-line resource reports a long list of symptoms which have been correlated with aspartame use; some of these which are also associated with chronic fatigue and fibromyalgia are listed in Table 20. Many people report improvement or disappearance of many symptoms when they discontinue use of aspartame products. Individuals who use these products and who have several of these symptoms are recommended to discontinue using aspartame for a period of thirty to sixty days to determine which, if any, of their symptoms improve.

Table 20. Reported Symptoms of Aspartame Consumption

Body System	Reported Symptoms
Cardiac	Chest pain, tachycardia, hypertension
Musculo-skeletal	Joint pains, muscle spasms, arthritis
Gastrointestinal	Abdominal pain, diarrhea, nausea or vomiting, weight gain
Hormonal	Blood sugar control problems (hypo-glycaemia or hyper-glycaemia), impotency and sexual problems, menstrual problems or changes
Neurological	Dizziness, hair loss or thinning of hair, flushing of face, hearing loss, hives (urticaria), anxiety attacks, numbness or tingling of extremities, seizures and convulsions, slurring of speech, tremors, tinnitus, vertigo, vision loss, excessive thirst or hunger, migraines and severe headaches, insomnia
Respiratory	Asthmatic reactions, chronic cough, laryngitis
Immune System	Chronic fatigue, infection susceptibility
Mood, personality	Confusion, depression, inability to concentrate, irritability, foggy thinking, memory loss, panic attacks, anxiety

Acutherapy to Boost Immune Functioning

Chong Mai/ Yin Wei Mai Extraordinary Vessels

Traditionally, the Chong Mai is said to arise from the Kidneys. According to Low (1983) the symptomology of this vessel suggests that the most likely site of origination is actually the adrenals. The Chong Mai connects several of the endocrine glands, including the gonads, adrenals, thymus, and thyroid. The Yin Wei Mai vessel is associated with the hormonal system through its point Ren-22 which is located near the thyroid gland. Yin Wei also has a connection to the Vagus Nerve through its points Ren-22, Liver-14, Spleen-13, Spleen-15, and Spleen-16. This vessel pair can be a powerful way of working with immune function because of this close association to the adrenals and endocrine system.

The acupoints for activating the Chong-Yin Wei connection are Spleen-4 and Pericardium-6. These may be worked in a variety of different ways, including acupressure, simple needling, needles with ion pumping cords, magnets (North pole against the skin on SP-4, South on PC-6), or ion pellets (Gold on SP-4, Silver, Copper, or Zinc on PC-6). Polarity agents such as magnets can be taped onto the points for the duration of the session. Clinical magnets may be up to 3000 gauss for in-office use. For home use, clients can be taught to use 600 or 800 gauss magnets which can be left on the points each night while sleeping. Practitioners who are not familiar with the use of magnets are recommended to take a course in magnet acutherapy or work with a practitioner who is knowledgeable about these techniques before using them with clients.

Ring of Fire Acutherapy

It has been suggested that DHEA is a biochemical analog of Qi, and a marker for the reserves of the adrenal glands (Shealy, 1996). Shealy has measured the DHEA levels of subjects before and after a series of acutherapy treatments using a group of twelve acupuncture points which he calls the "Ring of Fire," named for the Kidney Fire functions related to the adrenal glands.

Shealy found that the DHEA levels in the healthy test subjects were raised by stimulating these points using a gigaTens electrical stimulator, and he indicates that acupuncture needle treatment on the points is also beneficial. The points used in this study are listed below and illustrated in Diagram 5.

- Kidney-3 (bilateral): Source point and Earth point for Kidneys
- Ren-2 (more practical to use than Ren-1)
- Ren-6: Sea of Qi; tonifies both yin and yang
- Ren-18: On the sternum
- UB-23 (bilateral): Back-Shu point of Triple Burner
- PC-6 (bilateral): Connecting-Luo point of Pericardium, Master Point of Yin Wei Mai extra vessel
- LI-18 (bilateral): Windows of the Sky Point
- Du-20: Hundred Meeting point; most Yang point on the body

This is a very interesting combination of points. Shealy believes it creates an electrical circuit which activates the connection between the gonads, adrenals, thymus, and pituitary glands, and the Kidneys of Chinese medicine, and, through the Windows of the Sky point, activates the body-mind connection. Shealy reports having excellent results using the Ring-of-Fire treatment points on ill individuals also. If he is correct in his hypothesis that DHEA is a biological analog for Qi, and this treatment increases DHEA, then this group of acupoints may be extremely valuable for treating immune-suppressed individuals with chronic illness such as fibromyalgia and chronic fatigue syndrome. The author stimulates the Ring-of-Fire points by acupressure, magnets, and gold magraine and clients report feeling much more energized for several days after the sessions. Acupuncturists and acupressurists are encouraged to work with these points with their clients who are immune suppressed.

Diagram 5. Ring-of-Fire Acutherapy Points

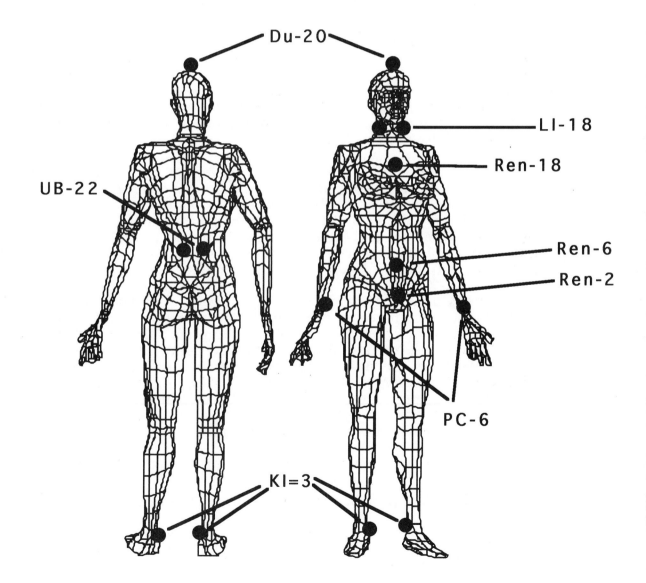

Chapter 9

Using the Lymphatic System for Fibromyalgia and Chronic Fatigue

OVERVIEW OF THE LYMPHATIC SYSTEM

The lymphatic system is one of the most under-appreciated and therapeutically under-used aspects of human physiology. This system is studied in every basic anatomy and physiology course in universities, medical schools, massage schools, acupuncture and chiropractic colleges, yet many health care practitioners do not yet recognize its importance or utility in working with chronic health problems. Most clients are not even aware of its existence or what they can do to improve it.

Functionally, the lymphatic system is part of the immune system and part of the circulatory system. Lymphatic fluid is essentially blood plasma, the clear fluid component of blood. It travels out of the circulatory system through the capillaries and into the interstitial spaces, carrying protein, antibodies, hormones and other materials into direct contact with the cells. The lymphatic fluid gathers waste products and cellular debris, and returns them to the circulatory system by the lymphatic vessels.

The lymphatic system can be effectively stimulated by massage or acutherapy. Acupuncture needles or hands-on massage techniques can be used with excellent results. There are trainings offered throughout the world in manual lymphatic drainage massage (MLD); these courses give in-depth theory and technique for the practitioner who wants to take advantage of the therapeutic leverage offered by the lymphatic system. In this chapter a general protocol for lymphatic stimulation will be presented, as well as acupoints and reflex areas which can be used in the clinic or at home by clients to improve immune functioning.

Possible consequences of poor lymphatic movement include:

- Failure of protein removal leads to edema, or swelling.

- Increased interstitial spaces moves cell walls a greater distance from their capillaries, affecting cellular nutrition and oxygenation.

- Sub-clinical functional impairment of tissue begins.

- Edema stretches the tissue, and can become chronic. Elasticity of the tissue diminishes, and increased permeability allows fluid accumulation to occur more easily.

- Sluggish movement gives greater tissue exposure to toxins and metabolic waste products, contributing to poor physiological performance, immune challenge, fatigue, and chemical sensitivity.

- Excess fluid accumulation is not clinically observable until it is approximately 30% above normal. Thus, lymphatic stagnation may be present long before it is observable to the client or practitioners.

- Maintenance of low-grade chronic infections of bacteria, fungal, or viral origin may be more likely.

- The immune system responds poorly to challenges from externally contacted virus, fungal, or bacterial pathogens.

- Continuous pressure on sensory nerve receptors in the edematous tissues can give rise to chronic discomfort, pain, and impaired muscle strength.

COMPONENTS OF THE LYMPHATIC SYSTEM

Components of the Lymphatic system are summarized here and shown in Diagram 6.

Capillary And Lymph Vessel Network For Transporting Lymph

The larger of these contain one-way valves to prevent back-flow. Movement through the vessels is facilitated by muscular contraction. There is no pump for the lymphatic system as the heart pumps the blood.

Lymph Nodes Which Collect And Filter Lymph

These are each about the size of a small kidney bean and occur in groupings near major veins. They perform a "straining" process on the lymph, and develop antibodies and lymphocytes if micro-organisms are present. When the system is working well, this process neutralizes harmful micro-organisms. The nodes become swollen when there is infection in their area of drainage, or when there are cancer cells spreading through the lymphatic vessels.

Cysterna Chyli

This structure is the pooling area for the lymph from the lower half of the body, including legs and abdominal area. It is located in the abdomen anterior to lumbar vertebrae 1 and 2.

Tonsils, Spleen, Thymus

These organs produce lymphocytes (white blood cells) which are vital to the immune system.

Lymphatic Fluid

This contains plasma proteins: gathers cellular waste products and debris, bacterial, and other particles from the interstitial spaces and returns all this to the bloodstream. Flow is upward against gravity, at rate of about three quarts per twenty-four hours.

Thoracic Duct

This is the major drain for most of the body, including all the lower body (it arises from the cysterna chyli), and the left side of the upper body; empties into the left subclavian and internal jugular veins.

Right Lymphatic Duct

This is the drain for the right upper half of the body and empties into the right subclavian and internal jugular veins.

Diagram 6. Components of the Lymphatic System

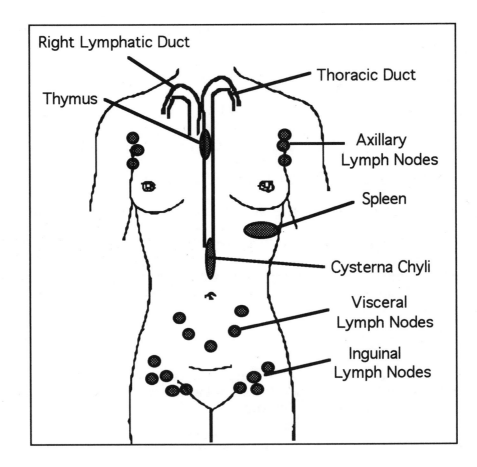

When doing lymphatic therapy, several of these areas correspond to the main lymphatic drains which are opened and cleared during the work. The drains are at the locations of the two lymphatic ducts at the clavicles, the axillary nodes, the cysterna chyli, and the inguinal nodes. Diagram 7 shows the locations of these drains on the body, and Diagram 8 is a schematic diagram showing the general pathways of lymphatic drainage in the body.

LYMPHATIC "DRAINS" AND LYMPHOTOMES

Lymphatic drainage work involves following the anatomical locations of lymphatic tissue and the natural drainage regions on the surface of the client's body. By doing this, the lymph can take the path of least resistance. Lymphatic work entails facilitating physical movement of a fluid through a slightly resistant medium. A skilled therapist can learn to feel and see the changes in the tissues and the fluids they hold.

Diagram 7. Lymphatic Drains Used in Therapy

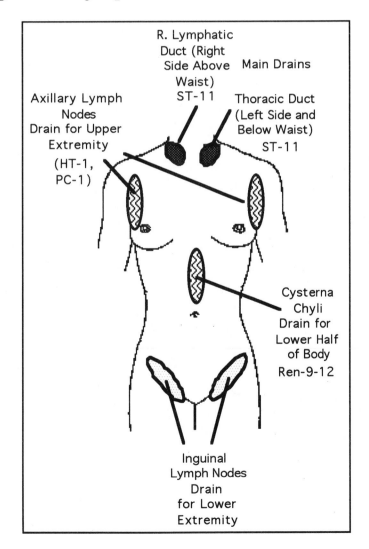

The lymphatic system is quite analogous to the drainage system in geographical areas on the earth's surface. Rain which falls on a certain area drains in a predictable direction into streams, which merge into larger rivers. Rivers eventually flow into the sea, where all the water converges. The body's lymphotomes work the same way; lymph in a particular lymphotome drains toward a specific lymphatic structure. Lymphotomes are separated by boundary lines, just as geographical drainage areas may be separated by a mountain range or other physical feature on the earth's surface. The boundary lines are called "water-sheds".

The illustrations in this chapter show the locations of the main lymphatic drains. During a lymphatic session, the drains will be used at the beginning, the end, and at intervals while the session is being conducted. The "drains" are locations where lymphatic material converges and is then transported to another location.

The main drains for the lymphatic system are at the medial ends of the clavicles, just superior and deep to the bones. All the lymphatic fluid of the body eventually moves into these drains, which empty into the subclavian and jugular veins and are then recirculated into the blood-circulatory system. Other important drain areas are at the Cysterna Chyli and at the locations where the limbs unite with the torso. The axillary and inguinal areas are rich with lymph nodes which filter all the lymphatic material returning from the extremity to the body cavities.   These locations of lymph nodes protect the vulnerable internal organs from possible infectious agents which may be acquired through injury or infection in the extremities.

Lymphotomes are regions in which lymphatic material flows in a characteristic predictable direction.   A metaphor may help the reader understand how the lymphotomes work. Visualize snow falling on the roof of a house. Snow evenly covers all the sloped surfaces of the roof. When the snow melts, the water flows in a particular direction, governed by the angle of the roof and the gravitational field, seeking it's lowest level. The water will never flow uphill and over the ridge of the roof to go down the other side.

The lymphotomes behave in a similar manner. Fluid within one lymphotome flows along its path of least resistance, and will not cross over into another drainage region in normal circumstances. When doing lymphatic drainage work, we want to respect these natural surface regions of the body and assist the fluid to move in its natural pathways. Careful study of Diagrams 9a through 9d will help the practitioner become familiar with the lymphotomes of each body region. It is recommended to work with only one area at a time initially, until you have become familiar with these drainage patterns.

Diagram 8. Schematic Diagram of Lymphatic Drainage

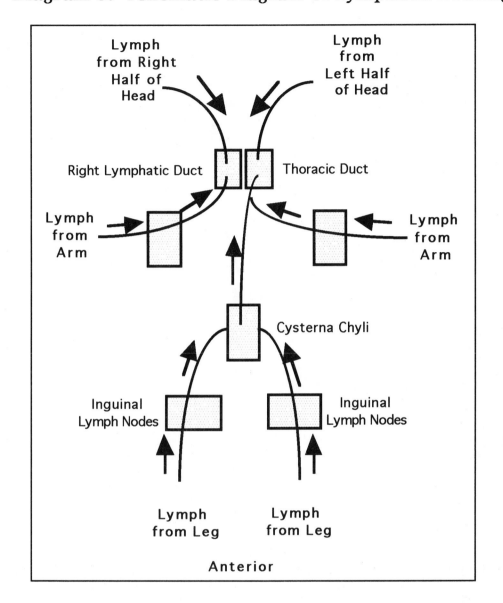

Lymphotomes of the Head (Diagram 9 a)

Each half of the head drains separately. From the mid-saggital line, all the superficial lymph of the face and scalp drains to the area at the angle of the jaw. From there, all the lymph flows downward in the neck, and empties directly into the main drains. The top of the shoulders above the clavicles and above the spinous processes of the scapulae also drains directly into the axillary nodes.

Diagram 9 a. Lymphotomes of the Head

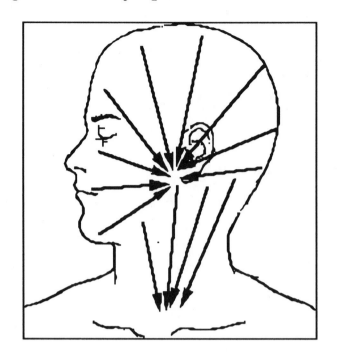

Lymphotomes of the Torso (Diagram 9 b)

Each half of the front and back torso drains as a mirror image of the other half. Regions above the waist drain to the axillary nodes, and regiions below the waist drain to the inguinal nodes. Lymph from the gluteal and sacral regions moves laterally around to the front. Lymph from the anal and genital areas drains anteriorly between the legs to the inguinal nodes.

Lymphotomes of the Upper Extremity (Diagram 9 c)

Lymph from the arms and hands drains into the axillary nodes in the region of Ht-1 to PC-1 (Diagram 9 c). All the lymph from the hand and forearm drains into the nodes in the antecubital area of Lu-5, PC-3, and Ht-3. The back of the upper arm (triceps) drains around to the front and joins the fluid moving upward from the forearm.

Lymphotomes of the Lowerr Extremity (Diagram 9d)

Lymph from the feet and legs drains into the inguinal nodes (Diagram 9 d). All lymph from the lower legs is filtered through the popliteal nodes in the back of the knee (KI-10, UB-54, UB-55). Lymph from the hamstrings travels to the front, joining the lymph of the quadriceps and the lower leg.

Diagram 9 b. Lymphotomes of the Torso

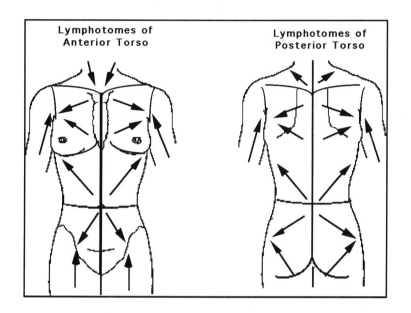

Diagram 9 c. Lymphotomes of the Upper Extremity

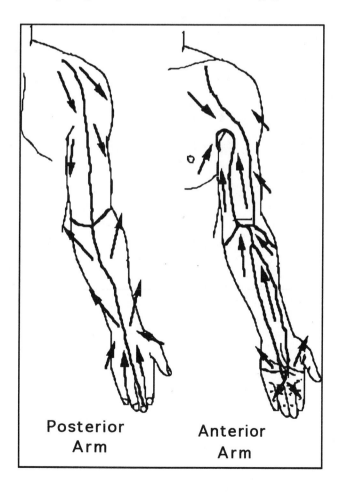

Diagram 9 d. Lymphotomes of the Lower Extremity

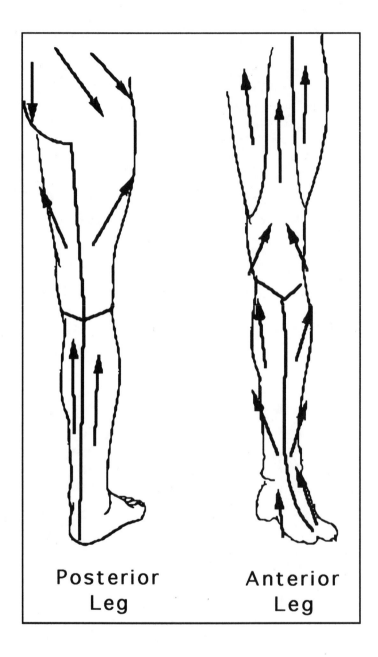

Posterior
Leg

Anterior
Leg

LYMPHATIC TECHNIQUES FOR ORIENTAL BODYWORK

Exercise 1. Developing "Lymphatic Touch"

Pressure for lymphatic work is very light, on the order of grams rather than ounces. Most therapists who are used to working with shiatsu, tuina, acupressure, or massage techniques are surprised when they feel how light the pressure is. Begin to familiarize yourself with lymphatic pressure by doing the following experiments. Touch your index finger to the back of your opposite hand and apply a little pressure. Observe the color of your nail bed; pressure should be light enough that the color remains unchanged. If the nail bed whitens, the pressure is too much. Using the correct pressure, move the finger without breaking contact with the skin, and notice how you can move the skin and underlying fascia a short distance. You can visually observe the changes in the skin texture as you gently stretch it.

Practice this exercise for a few minutes to get the feel of it. Touch several different places and notice how the skin may have varying tautness or slackness in different areas. Try the forehead, cheeks, throat, back of neck, and palm. Practice using both hands. Observe the slight stretching sensation you feel in the superficial tissues of the area being touched. This stretching sensation is an important marker for correct pressure; when doing lymphatic work, the receiver should be able to notice this. Spend a few moments working with longitudinal stretching, transverse stretching, and rotational movements on the surface of the skin. Pressure should not be at the depth of muscle tissue. Next practice applying this contact with two fingers side-by-side and with your full palm. Practice on several areas of the body surface, noting differences in tissue tension and puffiness.

With a little practice you can learn to feel the lymphatic congestion, or Dampness, in the tissues. It will feel soggy, boggy, spongy, puffy, moist, or thickened. Many times you can visually observe puffiness or pitting of the tissue. When the edema is even more severe an area may appear swollen, with bony landmarks such as the ankle bones being obscured; slight pressure may leave an indentation for a few moments.

The procedure given in this chapter should be done in a modular fashion. Select one or two areas of the body to work with in each bodywork session. Lymphatic work can bring on detoxification reactions which can be very uncomfortable for the client if too much work is done at one time. Instruct the client to drink adequate spring water or filtered water for a day or two after each session. A salt bath in the evening can also assist the body discharge. "Contrast hydrotherapy" is another method for stimulating the lymph system. At the end of a shower, make the water as cold as possible for thirty seconds, then hot for thirty seconds, and again cold for the last thirty seconds. Skin brushing after this gives a strong stimulation.

Summary of Hand Techniques for Lymphatic Bodywork

1. Light pumping

This is the technique for working the individual drains at the throat, cysterna chyli, axilla, and inguinal regions.

Exercise 2: Light Pumping on the Main Drains

Practice on yourself initially. Lie down in a comfortable supine position as if you were the client on a treatment table. Starting with the main drains, place your index and middle fingertips side-by-side in the soft areas just superior to the medial ends of the clavicles (**acupoint ST-11**). With light touch as practiced above, press into the soft tissue and caudally (toward the feet) slightly. Press rhythmically with slight twisting motion, approximately one press per heartbeat; you should be able to feel the slight changes in fluid pressure as you work. Pump ten to twenty times.

Next go to the axillary areas. Position your arm so that the axilla and the **Heart-1** and **Pericardium-1** acupoints are available; reach across with your opposite hand, and use two or three fingertips side-by-side. Lightly press into the axillary area, pumping with the same rhythm used at the main drains of the throat. Repeat for the other side. Again, you should feel the slight fluctuations in fluid pressure in the area. The goal is to pump excess fluid from the axillary nodes toward the main drains.

Next pump the cysterna chyli area at Ren-12, halfway between the umbilicus and the xiphoid process. Use palm-over-palm contact, to pump lightly into the belly and superiorly toward the head. The goal is to propel lymph up and out of the cysterna chyli toward the main drains. The last area is the inguinal node region. Place your hands on the inguinal creases, and lightly pump upward to propel the lymph from the legs toward the cysterna chyli.

2. Full-hand Fascial Stretching

Make full contact with your whole hand: palms, fingers, and thumb. Meld your hand lightly to the surface of the body so that when you move your hand, the skin and superficial fascia which contain the lymphatic capillaries are induced to move along with your hand (Review Exercise 1). Visualize a thin layer of adhesive or glue between your hand and the body, so that even slight pressure or movement can maintain the contact. Movements are small, and the receiver should feel a slight stretching sensation under the area of contact. Do this technique with respect to the lymphotomes. Practice on your own thigh, arm or chest areas.

When working along a lymphotome start at the end closest to the lymphatic "drain" and work distally. Pump approximately one press per heartbeat. You will usually be using both hands in one of two ways: 1) each hand in a different, but adjacent lymphotome, stretching in the respective directions of lymphatic drainage or 2) one hand stabilizing tissue upstream to the area where the other hand is doing the fascial stretching.

3. Vigorous Pumping

This is done with the same full-hand contact to the tissues, respecting the lymphotomes. Stay in one spot and apply a very light pressure (on the order of a few ounces of pressure), releasing pressure while still maintaining contact with the surface so that the tissue "rebounds". When working along a lymphotome, start at the end closest to the lymphatic "drain" and work distally. For example, on the arm start with the upper arm, then move to the forearm, then lastly work the hand.

This technique is used to strongly stimulate lymph-processing organs, such as liver and spleen, and at the ankles to propel lymphatic fluid up towards the torso. With the working hand, make full hand contact with the area to be pumped. Place "support" hand or "mother" hand underneath the body so your two palms are facing each other with the client's body in between. The hand on top will apply vigorous pumping, 2-3 pumps per second, to give an oscillating movement allowing the body to rebound each time. Your hand does not lift off but retains steady secure contact. There is a rolling component to the movement, which you achieve by slight rotation of your wrist and pronation of your forearm. For liver and spleen, direct your oscillations toward the navel.

4. Meridian Fascial Stretching

The subcutaneous fascia is the conduit through which the superficial meridians flow. By doing subtle fascial stretching, the therapist can open the meridian pathways and facilitate flow of Qi within them. If you are not yet familiar with the pathways, have a good meridian chart available in your work area. Select two contact points on the target meridian. These may be specific acupoints or they may be ah-shi points, or places which feel abnormal (tight, ropy, empty, gritty, squishy, gummy, hot, cold, tingly, etc.). Use fingertip or thumb pressure on each of your selected spots, and move one of your two contacts further away from the other to lengthen the meridian in that region. Even with very slight pressure (a few grams) you should be able to feel the pulling effect at your other contact. If you can't, select two points which are closer together, even as close as an inch or two apart. Work with gentle longitudinal stretching until you can feel a response at one contact point when you stretch the other. Gradually increase the distance between your two contacts, working small sections of the meridian at until you have opened up a long pathway.

5. Stretching Rotation

This is a variation of the simple meridian stretch described in #4 above. It is especially applicable for the arm meridians because they are short enough for the therapist to easily reach the whole length, and the arms have the pronating/supinating motion of the forearm. Establish a stationery contact on a point of the meridian on the torso (e.g. Lu-1, LI-16). Then grasp the arm at the wrist, with a firm contact on a distal point (e.g. Lu-9 or LI-4). Apply gentle traction to the limb while simultaneously pronating/supinating the client's forearm a bit to give a slight torquing-stretching action to the meridian.

TREATMENT PART I. CLIENT IN SUPINE POSITION

Opening The Major Lymphatic Drains By Light Pumping

To open the lymphatic drains, apply light pumping to the areas below in the order listed below. Pump each drain twelve to fifteen times at a rate of approximately twelve presses per minute.

- Thoracic duct and right lymphatic duct: <u>ST-11</u> area bilaterally
- Axillary nodes: <u>HT-1</u> area bilaterally
- Cysterna Chyli: <u>Ren-9 to 13</u> area
- Inguinal nodes: <u>ST-29, ST-30, Liv-12, Liv-13, Sp-13</u> area, bilaterally

Repeat this sequence at the beginning of every section. At the end of each section clear the drains by doing this sequence in reverse order.

Treatment For Anterior Upper Body

1. Therapist is positioned at client's head with palms over upper ribs. Apply full hand fascial stretching from sternum and Kidney points laterally toward the axillary nodes. Apply light pumping over the lung area to improve oxygenation.

2. With palms flat on the table, slide your hands and forearms underneath client's upper arms and place palms along lateral rib cage in the area of **SP-21, GB-22 and GB-23**. Do full hand fascial stretching and light pumping toward the axillary nodes.

3. Move to client's right side. Do palm-pressure shiatsu along the edge of the opposite rib margin to give stretching action. This helps release the diaphragm.

4. Place right hand underneath client's right ribs, and left hand on top of ribs. Pump the liver vigorously 50 times. Angle of pressure is toward navel.

5. Move to client's left side. Do palm-pressure shiatsu along the edge of the opposite rib margins to release second side of ribs and diaphragm.

6. Place your left hand underneath client's left ribs, and right hand on top of ribs. Pump the spleen/pancreas area vigorously 50 times. Angle of pressure is toward navel.

7. Repeat the opening movements at the major lymphatic sites. Working these areas periodically throughout the treatment assists the body to move the congested/stagnant lymph as you work.

Treatment For The Upper Extremities

1. The therapist is positioned by client's left side to treat the left arm first. Place left hand over the neurolymphatic area in the area of <u>LU-1 and LU-2,</u> at the front of the humerus, with medium pressure. Grasp client's wrist with your right hand in such a way as to press <u>LU-9</u> with your thumb, and then stretch the arm and do stretching rotation, stabilizing the shoulder and remaining within client's range of comfort. The client should feel a slight stretching sensation along Lung meridian.

2. Move your left hand to the middle of the sternum, with heel of palm near <u>Ren-14</u> area and front of palm over <u>Ren-17</u>. Apply medium pressure. Shift your right hand so you are now pressing <u>PC-7 and Ht-7</u> and repeat stretching rotation to stretch Heart and Pericardium meridians. Do this also with your left hand pressing the axillary region and stretching the meridians.

3. Move your right hand to the area of the acromion process of the scapula and lightly press <u>LI-16</u>. Grasp client's hand so you are pressing <u>LI-4</u> between your left thumb and forefinger and do a series of stretching rotations by circumducting the extended arm.

4. Holding the client's left wrist with your right hand, use your left hand and start the next series of movements on the YIN surface of the arm, on LU, PC and HT meridians near the axilla. Open the arm out and upward to expose this surface and apply full hand fascial stretching. Apply six presses at each area as you move distally. Your movement should be directed toward the axilla; visualize wringing a thick viscous fluid out of the arm toward the axillary nodes.

5. Next do the YANG surface of the arm, starting near the scapula and working distally toward the wrist in a similar manner as before.

6. Apply thumb pressure over the palm and back of the hand.

7. Use light wiping strokes over the whole length of the arm, following the lymphotomes toward the axillary nodes.

8. Repeat all steps for the right arm. Then work all the lymphatic areas again,as at the start of the routine.

Treatment For The Head And Neck

1. Therapist sits at client's head. Begin to work the neck and head area by doing palm and thumb pressing movements across the traps from medial to lateral and posterior to anterior. The lymph from this area drains directly into the thoracic duct on the left and the right lymphatic duct on the right. Angle the pressure movements toward these areas near <u>ST-11</u>.

2. Drain the neck by doing bilateral grasping pressing movements, starting at the C-7, T-1 level, and working up to the Occiput. This is a variation of fascial stretching in which you use both hands to encircle the neck. The thumbs lightly touch the posterior of the neck at the midline. The index fingers of both hands are in light contact with the sides of the receiver's neck, contacting the sternocleidomastoid muscles. Work slowly and deliberately, applying 6 to 8 presses at each level, and paying special attention to the sternocleidomastoid muscle. Direct your pressure toward the ducts. Repeat two or three times. Draining the neck and head can give much improvement for client's cognitive abilities, helping them to feel more clear headed.

3. Mobilize the neck vertebrae by placing your fingertips under the occipital bone (**Du-16, UB-10, and GB-20**), cradling the back of the head in your two hands, and then lift the head to flexion (chin toward the sternum). Go slowly and tell client to say "when" if you cannot feel when the stretch has gone far enough. Slowly lower the head back to the table as you simultaneously tilt it backward into extension (client's chin tips toward the ceiling). Your fingertips in the suboccipitals act as a fulcrum around which the occipito-atlantal joint can move. Repeat this motion smoothly 6 to 12 times.

4. Do deep circular massage on the suboccipitals.

5. Do deep pressing massage on the "Jade Pillow" (**BL-9**) area (external occipital protuberance) and along the mastoid process behind the ears, where Triple Heater meridian runs.

6. Do gentle pinching all along the jaw line, starting at the chin and moving toward the angle of the jaw. Direct your pressure toward the angle of the jaw, where all the lymph of the head and face collects before going to the major ducts. Be sure to get underneath the jaw bone also, and be very gentle. Many people have a good deal of congestion here, so it is often very tender. Repeat several times.

7. With your thumbs, do deep stroking across the forehead from the acupoint **Yin Tang** near the "third eye" laterally toward acupoint **Tai Yang** on the temples, and down toward the temperomandibular joint. Do 25 to 30 strokes, as time allows, giving thorough coverage of the forehead and temples. The strokes should be done slowly, and with enough pressure to leave a white streak as you go, showing that you are moving fluids of the skin and fascia.

8. Once again, work the major lymphatic areas around the throat, axilla, abdomen, and inguinal areas.

Treatment for the HARA (Abdomen)

Treatment of the Hara is very important for lymphatic work, as there are many lymph nodes all around the viscera. There are numerous excellent methods of treating the Hara in every style of Oriental Bodywork. You may use techniques you have already learned from shiatsu, Chi Nei

Tsang, TuiNa, Anma, or other modalities, or refer to the Hara treatment instructions in the general shiatsu treatment in this book (Chapter 11).

Treatment for the Anterior Lower Extremity

1. The front of the thigh is divided into three lymphotomes, center (over rectus femoris), medial and lateral. The Stomach and Spleen meridians approximate the boundaries of the lymphotomes on the anterior thigh. After light pumping the area of the inguinal nodes, start at the top of the thigh, and use two-hand fascial stretching for the center and medial lymphotomes. One palm lies within each lymphotome. Apply 6 to 8 stretches to each spot as you slowly move downward toward the knee. Then repeat, but this time using the center and lateral lymphotomes. When you reach the knee, gently pump the inguinal area again. If there is visible lymphatic congestion/ edema in the legs, repeat the work on the thigh at least one more time.

2. Use meridian fascia stretching for each meridian of the anterior thigh. Suggested point combinations for each meridian are as follows:

   * GB-30 and GB-33
   * ST-31 and ST-34
   * SP-10 and SP-12
   * and LIV-10

3. Do light pressure round-rubbing on the medial and lateral sides of the knee joint and at the "eyes" of the knee.

4. Do medium-pressure wiping strokes from the knee up to the inguinal area.

5. Do two-hand fascial stretching from just below the knee down to the ankle. Apply 6 to 8 stretches at each spot and work slowly, visualizing that you are moving a thick viscous fluid.

6. Do meridian fascia stretching on the meridians of the lower leg.

   * ST-36 and ST-42
   * GB-34 and GB-40
   * SP-9 and SP-4

7. Repeat steps 1 through 6 for the other leg.

8. Lymphatic pumping technique: Sit at client's feet so you are comfortable and well-balanced. Grasp the ball of the foot and toes firmly, and move the foot to a dorsiflexed position to take the slack out of the calf muscles. Then apply longitudinal rhythmic dorsiflections (vigorous pumping) of the foot in such a manner to produce undulating motion in the abdomen. You should strive to do 80-100 per minute, and sustain evenly for one minute. If client is very toxic and ill, fifteen to twenty seconds is enough initially. This propels lymph up the legs very effectively.

9. Pump the major lymphatic areas again, especially the inguinal nodes and the **Ren-9** to 13 cysterna chyli area.

PART II. CLIENT IS IN PRONE POSITION WITH ARMS AT SIDES

Work the major lymphatic areas from the back side as follows:

Working at client's head:

1. Light pump the major ducts at <u>ST-11</u> area 6 or 8 times by sliding your fingertips under the front of the shoulders.

2. Abduct client's upper arms a bit, place your fingers in axillary region and light pump toward you 6 to 8 times.

Move to the side of the client:

3. Apply light pumping motions on the spine from Thoracic-11 to Lumbar-3.

4. Light pump the top of the hamstrings, near <u>UB-50</u> at the sit-bone with your palms.

Treatment for the Upper Back

1. Standing near the client's head, work the area around C-6 to T-2 by applying two hand fascial stretching movements over the traps from the center outward, and over the traps toward the main drains at <u>ST-11</u>. If client has puffiness and edema in this area (buffalo hump) spend extra time in this region. This is an area of lymphatic reflexes for the Kidneys, Spleen and Lungs.

2. Apply round-rubbing over both scapulae. Then work the shoulder area one side at a time, one hand cradling the head of the humerus and the other pushing toward the axillary nodes. As you work, mobilize the shoulder with the hand underneath. Stretch the fascia and visualize draining fluid from the shoulder toward the axilla.

3. Work the rhomboid area from client's head. Use your two forearms, one on each side of the spine, like a rolling pin from medial to lateral. Also use your forearms without the rolling motion to stretch the fascia outward from the spine.

4. Work the middle-burner area from bottom of scapula to waist one side at a time. Use forearm rolling toward the axilla, then give one-hand fascial stretching with one palm while the other stabilizes the spine. All movements toward axilla.

5. Apply medium pressure wiping movements over the upper back, directing the lymph toward the axilla; pay attention to the lymphotomes as you work.

6. Starting at the waist level, pinch each of the spinous processes as you move up to the neck area. Do this with client's breathing, holding each process for one to three breaths.

7. Work the major lymphatic areas as described above.

Treatment for the Lower Back and Hips

1. Stand next to the client's hips. Apply vigorous round-rubbing to the sacrum and lumbar area to stimulate the Kidneys and lower burner area.

2. Working one side at a time, do fascial stretching medial to lateral over the lumbar area. Use one hand to push while the other hand stabilizes the spine.

3. On the sacro-iliac joint apply small finger-tip round rubbing. If the sacrum and/or sacro-iliac joint area is swollen and puffy, you may use moxa on the area.

4. Working one side at a time, do fascial stretching medial to lateral over the gluteal area. Visualize moving fluid around to the front where the inguinal nodes are located.

5. Place one palm on the lower part of the sacrum, fingers pointing toward the head and heel of hand at Du-2. Apply longitudinal thrusting motions to mobilize the whole spine. The entire torso should be visibly oscillating in the longitudinal axis. Your movements should be 80-100 per minute, but only do this for half a minute or less.

6. Starting at the L-5 level, pinch each of the spinous processes as you move up to the ribs area. Do this with client's breathing, holding each process for one to three breaths.

7. Apply medium-pressure wiping strokes over the low back and hips, paying attention to the lymphotomes.

8. Gently pump the major lymphatic areas once again.

Treatment for the Posterior Lower Extremity

1. Take a position at approximately the level of the client's knees, so you can reach the distance from the sacrum to the ankles. Start at the top of the hamstrings near UB-50, and use two-hand fascial stretching. Apply 6 to 8 press-pushes to each spot as you slowly move downward toward the knee. Position your hands with regard to the lymphotomes. The Bladder meridians approximates the boundary of the lymphotomes on the posterior thigh. When you reach the knee, gently pump the UB-50 area again. If there is visible lymphatic congestion/ edema in the legs, repeat the work on the thigh at least one more time.

2. Gently pump the posterior of the knee.

3. For the calf, use two hand fascial stretching movements again. Apply 6 to 8 press-pushes to each spot as you slowly move downward toward the ankle. Position your hands with regard to the lymphotomes.

4. Do pinching-grasping along the Achilles tendon.

5. Apply thumb, palm or fist pressure to the plantar surface of the foot.

6. Do stretching movements for the deep rotators of the hip. Position yourself alongside the client at hip level. For the external rotators, stabilize the sacrum with one hand. Then grasp the ankle, flex the knee 90 degrees, and pull the ankle toward you. Hold 5-10 seconds. Repeat 4 to 6 times. For the internal rotators, abduct the femur about 45 degrees from the hip, stabilize the GB-30 area (Greater trochanter), flex the knee, and push the ankle medially toward the opposite knee. Hold 5-10 seconds. Repeat 4 to 6 times.

7. Perform a psoas stretch as follows: Flex the knee 90 degrees, Place your hand (the one closer to the feet) under the knee so the ankle rests against your shoulder. Place your other hand on the sacrum to stabilize the hips. Then lift the knee straight up toward the ceiling, extending the hip to give a stretch to the psoas muscle. Hold 5-10 seconds, then lower the leg back onto the table. Repeat several times.

8. Pump all the lymphatic drains (in reverse order) one last time.

9. Finish the treatment with chakra balancing, point holding, or other movement to create a polished ending to the session.

10. Thank client for allowing you to participate in the shared experience.

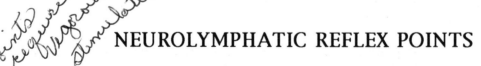

NEUROLYMPHATIC REFLEX POINTS

The neurolymphatic reflexes are points which stimulate the circulation of lymph. They can be worked in a massage or bodywork format or in an acupuncture session with needling. There are neurolymphatic reflexes for each of the twelve Organ-meridian circuits.

The neurolymphatic reflex areas should be palpated carefully to determine if they require stimulation. When distressed, they will be puffy, swollen, hardened, tense or tight, and tender to pressure. Shiatsu pressure or tuina movements can be applied with excellent results. These points require vigorous stimulation, as much as the client can receive, to stimulate movement. Apply circular massage for one to two minutes each. The client can be taught the locations for home massage.

It can be beneficial to spend an entire session just working the neurolymphatic reflexes. Have the client lie in the prone position and start working at the base of the neck. Refer to Diagram 10 and work all the reflex points along the spine to the sacrum. Note that the Bladder meridian accompanies these locations. Then have the client turn over, and work the front reflex points, starting at the upper ribs. Work down toward the Hara, and lastly work the areas on the inner and outer thighs. Note which areas are most pressure sensitive, and work the Source points and Front-Mu points for those Organ-meridians also. This makes an excellent treatment for individuals with fibromyalgia or chronic fatigue. The Neurolymphatic reflex points are illustrated in Diagram 10.

EXTERNAL APPLICATIONS TO PROMOTE THE LYMPHATIC SYSTEM

Castor Oil Packs

Benefits of Castor Oil Packs

Castor oil packs can be applied over the internal organs to eliminate toxins, promote lymphatic function, stimulate proper organ function, and many other benefits. Physiological effects of castor oil packs as identified by Edgar Cayce (Grady, 1988) include the following:

- Increase elimination
- Stimulate liver and gall bladder
- Dissolve and remove lesions, tumors and adhesions
- Relieve pain and inflammation
- Release colon impaction, stimulate cecum, reduce flatulence
- Reduce nervous system incoordination
- Reduce toxemia
- Increase systemic lymphatic circulation
- Improve nutrient assimilation
- Increase relaxation
- Reduce nausea
- Dissolve gall stones
- Reduce swelling
- Stimulate organs and glands
- Relieve headaches
- Stimulate peristalsis
- Increase blood and lymph circulation of the skin
- Draws acids (lactic acid, etc.) and infection out of tissues

Instructions for Castor Oil Packs

Gather the following items:

- Castor oil
- Cotton flannel fabric
- Terry cloth hand towel
- Heating pad

Purchase castor oil in a pharmacy where the laxative products are located. You will also need some cotton or wool flannel fabric which can be found in a fabric or sewing goods shop, or you can use an old flannel shirt or night-gown. Fold a piece of the fabric so it is about four layers thick and about the size of a wash cloth. Save the rest for another person, or for when you need to replace your cloth.

At bedtime, remove clothing and lie down on your back on your bed. Liberally apply castor oil to the area you wish to treat (usually colon, liver/gall bladder, or stomach/spleen/pancreas areas). Massage it in a bit to give good coverage. Place your folded flannel cloth over the area, and apply more castor oil between the layers of the cloth. Place the clean, dry hand towel over this to protect linens or bedclothes from being stained by the oil, and then place the heating pad on top of the towel. Cover up, and be calm and peaceful. Keep the heating pad as hot as you can to improve absorption and beneficial effects of the castor oil. Leave in place for a minimum of thirty minutes, and as much as ninety minutes. Turn the heating pad OFF before going to sleep. Cayce often recommended that castor oil packs be applied three nights in a row, then three nights off. This sequence is repeated for several weeks or even months in cases where chronic congestion and weakness is obvious.

Contrast Hydrotherapy

Contrast hydrotherapy can be done easily at home. At the end of a shower, the water is made as cold as possible. The person should stay in the cold water for thirty seconds to a minute, briskly rubbing the skin of the arms, legs, torso, and neck. Then make the water comfortably hot and stay for another thirty seconds to a minute, rubbing the body briskly. Then finally return the water to the cold setting for the last thirty seconds to one minute. Finish with a brisk rubdown with a towel. The alternating temperatures causes the lymph capillaries to contract, expand, and then contract again, pushing stagnant lymph along to be recirculated. This is very invigorating and can be done two to three times per week. Combine with skin brushing for an especially strong lymphatic work-out.

TRADITIONAL CHINESE MEDICINE AND THE LYMPHATIC SYSTEM

In traditional Chinese medicine the lymphatic system is included in the concept of Blood. Blood, for TCM, has a larger context than blood of Western medicine; it includes many body fluids in addition to the red blood of the circulatory system. Among the fluids it may include are blood, lymph, intracellular fluid, synovial fluid, interstitial fluid, menstrual blood, and digestive fluids. Most fluids of the body can be classified as "Blood" with the exception of seminal fluid and cerebrospinal fluid, which correspond more closely with the concept of Jing or Essence and the "special fluids" such as tears, urine, saliva, sweat, nasal mucus and so on.

[handwritten margin note at top: "DAMPNESS" produced by over work, excessive mental exertion or worry and obsessive thinking]

Stagnation or sluggishness of the lymphatic system corresponds to the Blood Stagnation patterns and Phlegm patterns defined by Chinese medicine, and by retention of the Damp pathogen in the body. In the case of lymphatic stagnation, Dampness is produced internally rather than as an External Pernicious Influence. Dampness arises primarily because of deficiency of Spleen-Qi. The most frequent causes of Spleen-Qi deficiency include over-consumption of simple sugars and starches; cold, raw, foods and drinks, overwork, and excessive mental exertion or worry and obsessive thinking. Spleen-Qi deficiency is a central imbalance for most individuals with fibromyalgia, and for many with chronic fatigue.

The muscle and joint pain of fibromyalgia is treated as chronic painful obstruction syndrome. This can arise from deficiency of Qi and Blood, or from Phlegm in the joints, Blood stagnation, or deficiency of Kidneys and Liver. Checking the pulses, Hara, tongue, and other assessment methods will help the practitioner decide which pattern is present. Strategies for acutherapy focus on increasing Spleen energy, helping the client learn changes that will allow the Spleen to heal, and elimination of the Damp pathogen. Table 21 summarizes therapeutic approaches to lymphatic congestion.

[handwritten margin note: joint & muscle pain can arise from Qi deficiency of Kidney & Liver]

Table 21. Therapeutic Approaches to Lymphatic Congestion

Acupoints to Tonify Spleen-Qi	Acupoints to Resolve Damp, Phlegm and Move Blood	Client Homework to Improve Lymphatic Functioning	Herbs, Supplements,
Spleen-3	Spleen-6	Eliminate refined sugar	4-day colon cleanse
Spleen-6	Stomach-36	Eliminate white flour	Ginger
Stomach-36	Stomach-40	Eliminate artificial sweetener	Poke root tincture
Liver-13	Spleen-9	Use only sea salt	Echinacea
Ren-12	Spleen-10	Avoid MSG and "hidden salt"	Burdock root
UB-20	Ren-4	Skin Brushing	Dandelion root
Ren-8 (moxa)	Ren-9	Mini-trampoline	Kava kava
Spleen-4	Stomach-25	Walking- Stretching	MSM
		Increase physical activity	Glucosomine
Moxa may be Used as long as no Heat signs are present	Moxa may be used as long as no Heat signs are present.	Lymphatic massage	Evening primrose oil
		Acutherapy	Dong Quai
		Consume adequate pure water	
		Contrast (cold-hot-cold) shower	
		Castor oil packs ()	

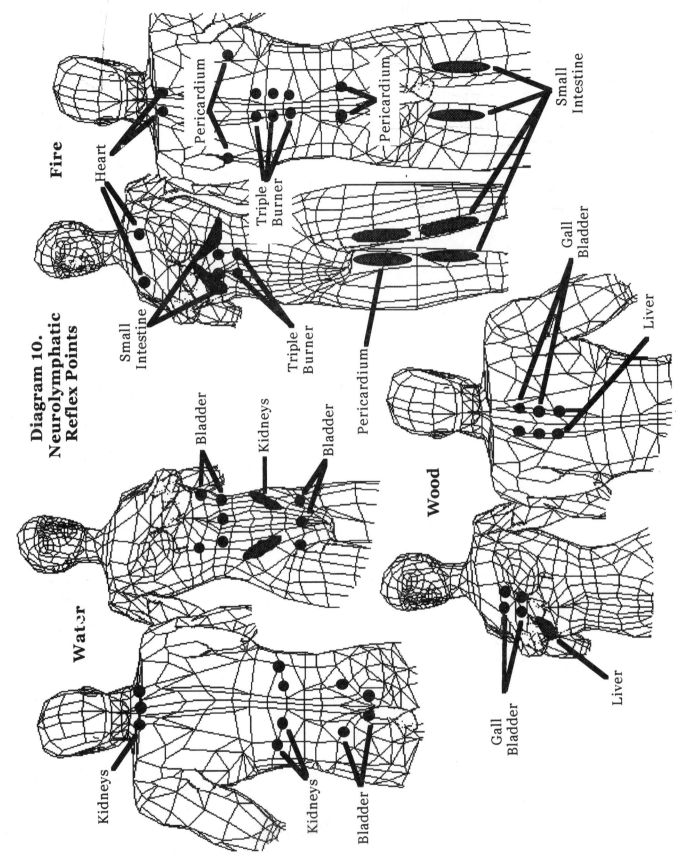

**Diagram 10.
Neurolymphatic
Reflex Points**

Fire

Heart

Pericardium

Pericardium

Small
Intestine

Small
Intestine

Triple
Burner

Small
Intestine

Triple
Burner

Pericardium

Water

Bladder

Kidneys

Bladder

Kidneys

Kidneys

Bladder

Wood

Gall
Bladder

Liver

Gall
Bladder

Liver

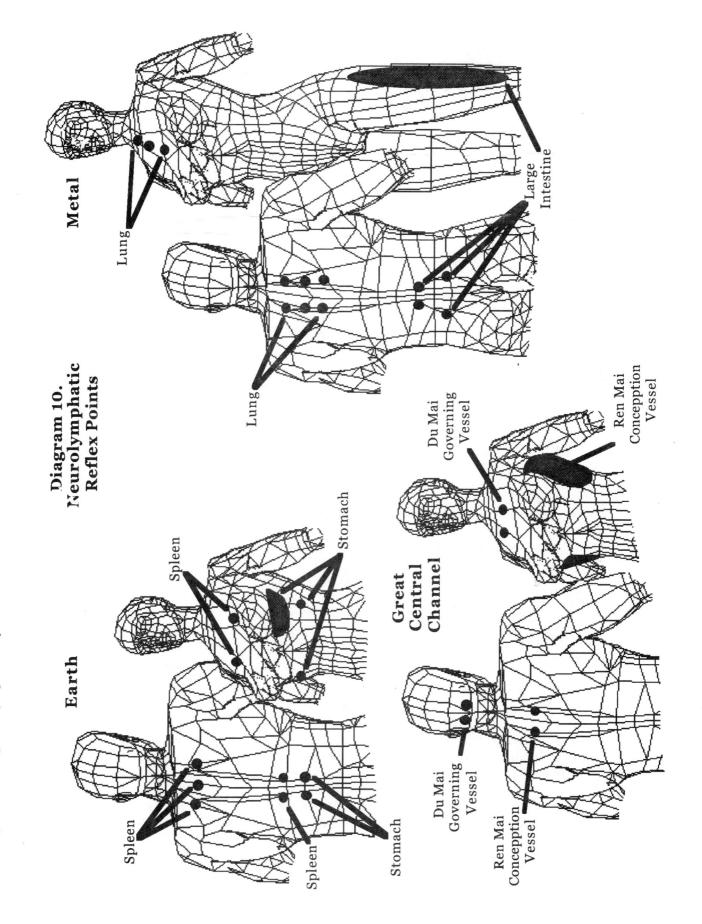

**Diagram 10.
Neurolymphatic
Reflex Points**

Metal

Lung

Lung

Large
Intestine

Earth

Spleen

Spleen

Spleen

Spleen

Stomach

Stomach

**Great
Central
Channel**

Du Mai
Governing
Vessel

Ren Mai
Concepption
Vessel

Du Mai
Governing
Vessel

Ren Mai
Concepption
Vessel

Chapter 10

Aromatherapy for Fibromyalgia and Chronic Fatigue Syndromes

INTRODUCTION TO AROMATHERAPY

Aromatherapy is the use of botanical essential oils for healing purposes. Numerous species of herbs, trees, flowers and shrubs produce essential oil, which has been described as the "blood" of the plant. The oils are extracted from the plants by several different methods, the most common of which is steam distillation.

The essential oils of many plants have been used in healing for centuries. There are numerous references to essential oils in the Bible, including frankincense, myrrh, hyssop, and spikenard. Modern studies have assisted researchers in understanding the mechanisms by which the essential oils can shift the body's chemistry. The same therapeutic actions are identified for essential oils as for herbs which are taken orally and for synthetic medications. Laboratory analysis has revealed the biochemical components which may account for the effectiveness of essential oils. Terpenes, sesquiterpenes, alcohols, phenols, ketones, esters and other classes of compounds have been isolated from plant essential oils. They are the same constituents that are believed to give medicinal herbs their therapeutic value. Some of the most important therapeutic properties for fibromyalgia and chronic fatigue are summarized in Table 22. Holistic practitioners are often more interested in the energetic effects of therapeutic agents than in the chemical components.

Essential oils can be administered in several ways. In the clinical setting they can be blended in a vegetable oil or cream base and applied to the skin. Essential oils are lipophilic, meaning they are attracted to fatty substances such as vegetable oil or the oil on human skin. Topical application is an excellent way to give local or systemic effect. The massage oil blend can be applied to the abdomen, spine, or soles of feet to give systemic effect, or they can be applied directly to the area of concern. Because they are extremely concentrated, essential oils should not be applied to the skin without a carrier oil. The carrier oil also helps the essential oils remain in contact with the skin longer because of their lipophilic properties. Excellent carrier oils include sesame, grapeseed, almond, and sunflower oil. Oil blends can be used in clinical sessions and by the client at home.

Essential oils can also be diffused into the treatment room or living area. An appliance called a diffuser can be purchased from essential oil vendors and massage supply companies for this purpose, or a few drops of essential oil can be placed on a tissue or cotton ball which is placed over a light bulb, so that the heat from the bulb volatilizes the oil. At night, a few drops can be applied to a cotton ball which is placed on a bedside table or in the client's pillow case. In these diffusion methods the oil is volatilized into the air and taken into the body by inhalation.

At home, the client can add a few drops of essential oil to hot bath water, in addition to the methods mentioned above. In the bath, the oils will be absorbed dermally and inhaled through the lungs. Blends designed to promote restful sleep or relieve muscular discomfort are especially effective ones to use in hydrotherapy. Essential oils should never be taken internally by mouth. When recommending oils to clients for home use, it is important to instruct them in the proper usage of a powerful therapeutic agent. Therapeutic quality essential oils are costly and only a very small quantity is needed for good results.

CHINESE MEDICINE AND AROMATHERAPY

Essential oils can be categorized according to their Five-Element correspondences, by their effects on the Vital Substances, and by their ability to affect Pernicious Influences. This is useful information for the acupuncturist or oriental bodywork therapist working with TCM assessment and treatment.

Table 23 summarizes several of the more commonly used essential oils by Five-Element categories. The oils listed for each element have the effect of nourishing or tonifying that element's energetic activities. When an element has been identified as deficient, the practitioner can select oils from the list for that element to strengthen the element. When an element has been identified as excess or overactive, the practitioner should select oils from the controlling element's list. The five-element relationships (control and creation cycles) are shown in Diagram 11.

Table 22. Therapeutic Properties of Essential Oils

Property	Definition	Essential Oils
Anti-bacterial	Destroys or inhibits bacterial growth	Bergamot, Cedarwood, Clary Sage, Clove, Geranium, Hyssop, Melaleuca, Oregano, Patchouli, Rosemary
Anti-catarrhal	Helps remove excess mucus	Cedarwood, Eucalyptus, Ginger, Helichrysum, Hyssop, Juniper, Myrrh, Rosemary, Sandalwood
Anti-depressant	Alleviates depression; lifts spirits	Bergamot, Clary Sage, Frankincense, Geranium, Jasmine, Lavender, Myrrh, Orange, Rose, Sandalwood, Vetiver, Ylang-ylang
Anti-infectious	Prevents the spread of infectious agents	Eucalyptus, Oregano, Pine, Rose, Spikenard
Anti-rheumatic	Helps relieve or prevent rheumatism	Birch, Cypress, Eucalyptus, Juniper, Lavender, Lemon, Pine, Rosemary, Thyme, Vetiver,
Anti-spasmodic	Prevents or eases spasms, cramps	Bergamot, Birch, Chamomile, Clary sage, Cypress, Geranium, Helichrysum, Lavender,Marjoram, Orange, Peppermint, Rosemary, Thyme, Vetiver, Ylang-ylang
Anti-viral	Inhibits the growth of viruses	Clove, Eucalyptus, Hyssop, Melaleuca, Myrrh, Peppermint, Ravensara, Sage
Analgesic	Reduces physical pain and discomfort	Birch, Chamomile, Eucalyptus, Frankincense, Geranium, Ginger, Lavender, Lemongrass, Marjoram, Peppermint
Immune stimulant	Promotes the body's natural defenses	Cinnamon, Frankincense, Eucalyptus, Hyssop, Lemon, Melaleuca, Oregano, Patchouli, Thyme
Calmative	Relaxes and calms the mind and body	Bergamot, Cedarwood, Cypress, Frankincense,Geranium,Helichrysum, Sandalwood, Ylang-ylang
Lymphatic decongestant	Assists movement of lymphatic material	Cypress, Geranium, Grapefruit, Juniper,Lemon, Sandalwood

Table 23. Essential Oils and the Five Elements

WATER	WOOD	FIRE	EARTH	METAL
Cedarwood	Bergamot	Ginger	Lemon	Clary Sage
Cypress	Chamomile	Rose	Patchouli	Cypress
Geranium	Helichrysum	Rosemary	Vetiver	Eucalyptus
Juniper	Grapefruit	Lavender	Sandalwood	Frankincense
Pine	Lavender	Marjoram	Orange	Hyssop
Birch	Lemon	Thyme	Myrrh	Pine
	Orange	Jasmine	Marjoram	Melaleuca
	Rose	Ylang-ylang	Ginger	Sandalwood
	Peppermint	Cinnamon	Clove	Oregano
			Ginger	
			Peppermint	
			Lemongrass	

Diagram 11. Five Element Creation and Control Cycle

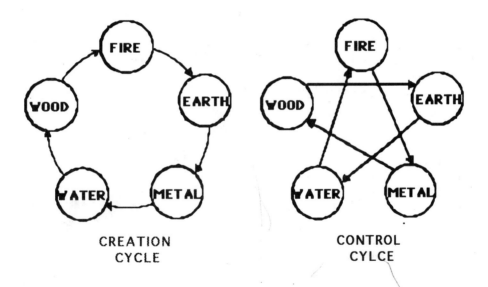

These essential oils can also be classified according to their effects on Qi and Blood and on External Pathogenic factors. Their effects are summarized in Table 24 and Table 25.

Table 24. Essential Oil Effects on Qi and Blood

Tonify Yang	Tonify Yin	Tonify Qi	Tonify Blood	Move Stagnant Qi	Move Stagnant Blood
Juniper Rosemary Thyme	Geranium Rose Vetiver Birch	Cedarwood Clary Sage Eucalyptus Geranium Ginger Hyssop Jasmine Lavender Marjoram Myrrh Patchouli Pine Melaleuca Ylang-ylang Oregano	Cypress Geranium Grapefruit Rose Ylang-ylang	Bergamot Chamomile Clary Sage Cypress Helichrysum Grapefruit Marjoram Orange Peppermint Rose Lavender	Lemon Helichrysum Rose Rosemary Pine

Table 25. Essential Oils and Pernicious Influences

Cooling (For Heat Patterns)	Warming (For Cold Patterns)	Dispels Damp (For Damp Patterns)	Moistening (For Dry Patterns)	Expels Wind (For Wind Patterns)
Bergamot Chamomile Helichrysum Geranium Lavender Lemon Peppermint Rose Sandalwood Ylang-ylang Birch Grapefruit	Cedarwood Ginger Hyssop Juniper Marjoram Myrrh Patchouli Pine Rosemary Thyme Cinnamon Clove Oregano	Cedarwood Eucalyptus Ginger Grapefruit Juniper Lemon Marjoram Myrrh Peppermint Pine	Geranium Frankincense Lavender patchouli Jasmine Myrrh	Chamomile Grapefruit Peppermint Eucalyptus Marjoram Ginger Helichrysum Thyme

Table 26. Essential Oils for Chronic Fatigue and Fibromyalgia Symptom Reduction

Immune Boosting	Relieve Fatigue	Alleviate Depression	Promote Sleep	Muscular Pain	Mental Clarity
Cinnamon Frankincense Melaleuca Myrrh Oregano Hyssop Patchouli Sandalwood Vetiver Lemon Thyme Clove	Cinnamon Cypress Juniper Peppermint Bergamot Lemon Clary Sage Lavender	Bergamot Chamomile Clary Sage Frankincense Grapefruit Helichrysum Lavender Lemon Marjoram Rose Melaleuca Orange Patchouli Peppermint Thyme Ylang-ylang	Clary Sage Lavender Geranium Vetiver Lemon Chamomile Orange	Birch Lemongrass Marjoram Eucalyptus Geranium Chamomile Helichrysum	Chamomile Clove Hyssop Lemon Rosemary Thyme Peppermint Juniper Lemongrass Ylang-ylang

BLENDING GUIDELINES

Making blends for aromatherapy which are effective and aesthetically pleasing is an art as well as a science. Essential oils can be classified according to their blending properties. The heaviest and longest-lasting aromas are called "base notes" and usually make up 5-10% of a blend. The lightest and most volatile oils are called "top notes" and make up another 5-10% of a blend. "Middle notes" are intermediate in their volatility, and make up the bulk of most blends, as much as 80%. Essential oils in their blending categories are summarized in Table 27.

Start with simple three-component blends. Select a base note, a middle note, and a top note from the tables in this chapter to give the desired effect. For example, if the Earth element is deficient, one might choose patchouli as a base note, lemongrass as a middle note, and peppermint as a top note. For experimenting, place the drops on a cotton ball in a small paper cup, let the blend "develop" for five minutes, and then inhale the aroma to evaluate

Use approximately five drops of the middle note and one drop each of the base and top notes. You may add a drop more of any of the components to adjust the blend, or when your feel confident, add a fourth component. Keep the cotton ball with the experimental blend in your vicinity for an hour or longer and notice how you feel. Also notice how the blend changes. When you have a synergy that is interesting and aesthetically pleasing, write down the formula. Make up more of the blend in a small glass vial or bottle and try it with clients. Palpate for changes in the pulses or Hara reactivity before and after applying the blend to evaluate its ability to create the desired energetic shifts. For massage oil blends use twenty to forty drops of essential oil per one   ounce of vegetable oil.   For diffusing or hydrotherapy applications, use essential oil without a carrier oil.

20-40 drops for 1 oz carrier oil

Table 27. Essential Oil Blending Categories

BASE NOTES	MIDDLE NOTES	TOP NOTES
Sandalwood	Chamomile	Lemon
Rose	Helichrysum	Peppermint
Pine	Geranium	Bergamot
Cedarwood	Lavender	Ylang-ylang
Ginger	Rose	Grapefruit
Jasmine	Birch	Juniper
Cinnamon	Cypress	Cypress
Patchouli	Rosemary	Thyme
Myrrh	Marjoram	Orange
Vetiver	Lemongrass	Clove
Clary Sage	Eucalyptus	
Frankincense	Hyssop	
Oregano	Melaleuca (Tea Tree)	

Formula { 1 drop base note   5 drops of middle note   1 drop of Top note

BLEND FORMULAS FOR CHRONIC FATIGUE AND FIBROMYALGIA

The following formulas may be beneficial for symptoms of fibromyalgia and chronic fatigue. Combine the number of drops of each oil to make one ounce of a massage oil aromatherapy blend.

Mental Clarity Formula

1	Clove
4	Peppermint
6	Lavender
8	Rosemary
2	Clary Sage
2	Ginger

In 1 ounce carrier oil. Apply to temples, forehead, throat, neck, or diffuse in room.

For Muscle Pain, Headache, or to promote mental alertness

10	Marjoram
20	Lavender
10	Peppermint

in 1 ounce carrier oil. Massage into areas of discomfort. For headache or mental alertness apply to temples, back of neck, shoulders, wrists, soles of feet.

Anxiety/ Depression Relief Blend

8	Cedarwood
10	Lavender
5	Sandalwood
5	Geranium
5	Ylang Ylang
10	Bergamot

In 1 ounce of carrier oil. Apply on soles of feet, spine, neck and shoulders, chakra points, wrists, and liver area to lift and calm the spirits. Do not apply to areas which may be exposed to the sun, as bergamot can cause skin discoloration upon exposure to the sun.

Muscle and Joint Pain

20	Birch
10	Lemongrass

in 1 ounce carrier oil
Use as a deep massage oil. Highly recommended for home use for the pain of fibromyalgia syndrome or arthritis. Apply and massage into areas of pain.

Immune Boosting Formula

3	Frankincense
6	Melaleuca (Tea Tree)
1	Clove
4	Hyssop
1	Thyme

In 1 ounce carrier oil. Apply to soles of feet, chest, throat, lower abdomen, or lumbar area.

Promote Restful Sleep

8	Lavender
3	Blue (German) Chamomile
2	Clary Sage
4	Orange

in 1 ounce carrier oil. At bedtime, massage on abdomen, neck, temples, wrists.

Lift Depression

3	Clary Sage
3	Bergamot
5	Lemon
10	Marjoram

In 1 ounce carrier oil. Apply to soles of feet, throat, wrists, neck, abdomen, spine.

Clear Lymph Nodes, Relieve Sore Throat

10	Citronella
10	Lavender
10	Lemongrass
5	Melaleuca (Tea Tree)
2	Clove

in 1 ounce of carrier oil.
Apply to neck and throat to relieve sore throat or swollen lymph nodes.

Menstrual Difficulties and PMS

3	Patchouli
10	Lavender
5	Clary Sage
2	Basil
10	Grapefruit

In 1 ounce of carrier oil. Massage into lower belly and low back to soothe menstrual difficulty. May be used between periods also.

Blend for Clearing Emotional Trauma

5	Rose
5	Helichrysum
5	Frankincense
10	Sandalwood
20	Lavender
10	Geranium

in 1 ounce of carrier oil. Apply to liver area, heart area, spine, soles of feet, neck and throat, chakra points. Helps mobilize repressed memories or emotions in a gentle way to allow them to be released, worked with, and healed.

Family members can use this Technique sequence

Chapter 11

Oriental Bodywork Treatment for Fibromyalgia and Chronic Fatigue

This chapter contains instructions for a full-body shiatsu therapy session. It is designed to be used by anyone who has the opportunity to work with a person who has fibromyalgia or chronic fatigue. Professional therapists may obtain new ideas and techniques for integrating with other methods they are already using. Family members or friends may also use this technique sequence. Many have learned to help their loved one with just this simple procedure. It feels wonderful to have the full body session performed. Those who have little or no experience administering massage or bodywork techniques can give a very effective treatment if you carefully watch and listen for your subject's responses. Communication is a vital part of a good therapy session.

The sequence as written here offers a full treatment which takes about one hour to complete if all steps are performed. For shorter sessions use just a few of the techniques and work on one or two trouble areas. Acupoints are specified for those who are already familiar with the points and meridians and for students learning them.

Treatment Goals: Diminish muscular discomfort, boost energy level and mood, facilitate restorative sleep.

Treatment Strategy: Tonify the Qi and Blood, resolve Dampness, and lead the receiver to a deep relaxed state of comfort and well-being.

Technique: When treating specific points, start with very gentle superficial pressure. Feel for a pulsing in the point which indicates a "release", and increase pressure gradually as you assist the area to release layer by layer. Ask the client to let you know about the comfort of your pressure. Watch the client's face for nonverbal cues about the comfort level of your work. Work with the client's breathing pattern as much as possible, applying pressure on the exhale and releasing on the inhale.

PART I: FRONT OF BODY

Treatment for Neck, Shoulders, Arms, Chest, Ribcage

Client is supine on treatment table or futon, therapist positioned at client's head. Instruct the client to let you know if your pressure is appropriate, or if she/he needs to change positions, or if the temperature in the room needs adjusting for greater comfort. Pressure should be in the receiver's comfortable range, up to a "good hurt". For many people who have fibromyalgia, very light pressure will be enough. Strive to make the session a pleasant and comforting experience.

1. Cradle the receiver's head in your two hands, with fingers touching points along the base of the skull occipital ridge BL-10, GB-20, TB-16). Lift your fingertips up slightly toward the ceiling, allow the weight of the receiver's head to rest on your fingertips (Figure 1). Hold 30-60 seconds or even longer if your hands are strong enough.   This will help relax the neck muscles and the whole spine.

2. Turn the head slightly toward one side, and apply gentle circular friction and/or pressure to the point GB-20. From there, work down the posterior and lateral aspects of the neck with gentle thumb pressure (Figure 2). Pause at any spots which are knotted, tight or sore, and just hold gentle pressure for a few moments until you feel a pulsing sensation in the point. Then turn the head to treat the other side of the neck in a similar fashion. There is frequently a great deal of stagnation in the neck and skull area in fibromyalgia. The receiver may feel a significant release after having this area treated, and will usually become much more relaxed.

Figure 1   **Figure 2**

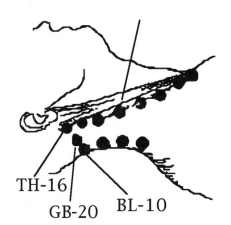

3. With the head in a neutral position, work systematically over the entire scalp area with circular pressure as firmly as the receiver can enjoy. For some individuals this will be very light, such as lightly shampooing a baby's hair; others will like extremely deep pressure. Adjust pressure to give a "good hurt" or less, and aim for thorough coverage without necessarily trying to follow the meridians or points. You may also treat the forehead in this manner, which will help to release points on the Stomach and Gall Bladder channels in that area.

   Next, work across the top of the shoulders, giving palm pressure to the trapezius muscles from the neck out toward the acromium (Figure 3). Key points in this area are GB-21 and LI-16. Hold gentle pressure on each bilateral pair for a moment or two. Both these points will get energy moving in the correct direction.

4. Slide your fingertips underneath the shoulder blades to get to TB-15 and SI-10 (Figure 4). Hold gentle pressure and/or circular pressure on each of these points. They may be very tender, so go slowly and gently.

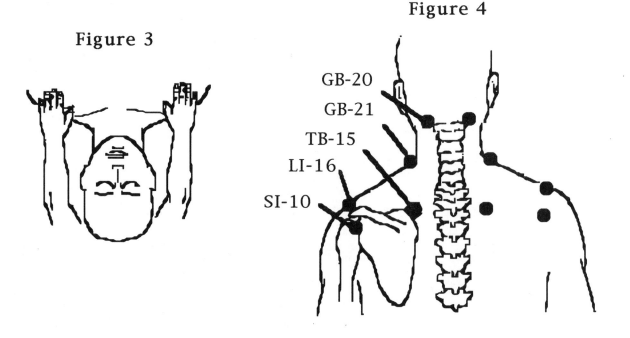

Figure 4

Figure 3

GB-20
GB-21
TB-15
LI-16
SI-10

5. Next move to the left side of the client to treat the left arm. On the Yin channels, work from the shoulder out toward the hand (Figure 5A). You may work all the channels together with palm pressure, or do them individually with thumb or finger pressure. Key points in this section are Lu-5 (resolves Upper Burner dampness), Lu-9 (Tonification point and source point for Lung), and PC-6 (lifts the spirit, restores proper direction of Qi flow, relieves anxiety, balances emotions) (Figure 5B). Hold each of these with gentle static pressure for 30-60 seconds.

6. Work the Yang channels of the left arm, from the hand toward the shoulder. These may be treated together with palm pressure, or individually with thumb or finger pressure. Key points in this section are LI-4, LI-11, TB-5 and TB-7 (Figure 6).

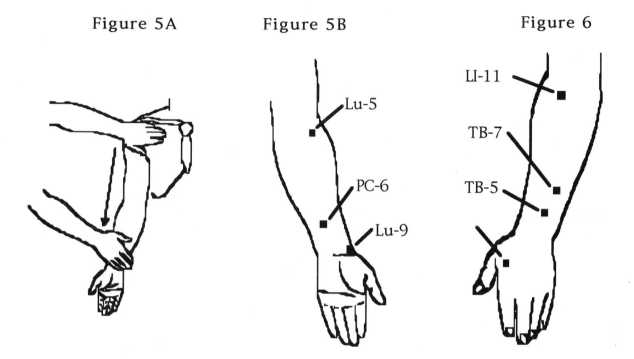

Figure 5A   Figure 5B   Figure 6

7. Next work the left shoulder blade. Sit or kneel facing the shoulder. Place your left hand (palm up) underneath the shoulder, and let your fingers press upwards into the muscles at the medial edge of the blade. On some people you will be able to hook your fingertips under the medial edge of the blade and gently pull toward you. Use your other hand to work with gentle finger or palm pressure on the front of the shoulder joint, (Figure 7). The hand beneath and the hand on top can work together in creative ways for a gentle joint mobilization for the shoulder joint.

Next place your top hand solidly on the side of the rib cage, and mobilize the ribs and diaphragm area by rocking the ribs laterally (push away from yourself while stabilizing the scapula with the hand underneath; then let the chest return to its neutral position. Perform for a minute or so, rhythmically). This is very effective for releasing the entire chest area, and people often find it easier to breathe after these techniques have been performed. Repeat steps 5, 6, and 7 for the right arm.

8. The next area includes the sternum and upper ribs. Begin with palm pressure, and place one hand on the client's sternum with your fingers pointing toward the head. Use gentle pressure to work from the bottom of the sternum up towards the sternoclavicular junction. Continue the palm

pressure laterally across the pectoral muscles and upper ribs, just below the collarbones. Make 4-5 trips up the sternum, alternately treating the right and left sides of the upper ribs (Figure 8). If the palm pressure is comfortable for the client, you may then switch to thumb or fingertip pressure. Be careful, as this is a sensitive area for many, and thumbs and fingers can feel more invasive. It may take several treatments with only palm pressure in this area before the client will be able to receive a more penetrating technique.

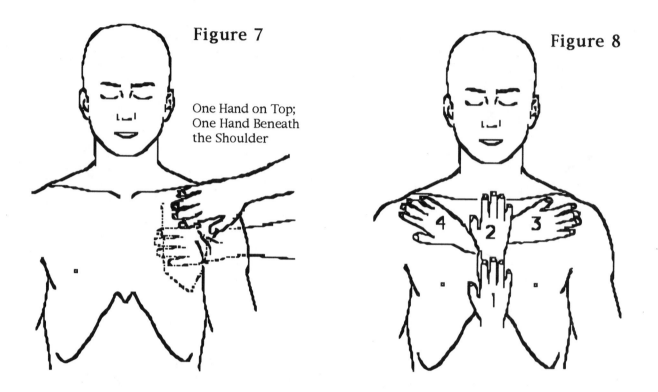

Figure 7

One Hand on Top;
One Hand Beneath
the Shoulder

Figure 8

Hara Treatment

9. The abdomen, or "Hara" as it is refered to in Japanese therapies, is an extremely important area to treat because it contains the internal organs. The intestines, kidneys, stomach, liver, female organs, and urinary bladder will all benefit from the increase in circulation, lymphatic movement, and energy flow from doing good Hara massage. Many people who have fibromyalgia have had multiple abdominal surgeries, and this part of the treatment can begin to release some of the stagnation which is often found in the belly after surgical interventions. Plan on spending a minimum of 5-10 minutes in this area during the treatment. Hara shiatsu does not need to be complicated; repetition of simple techniques for the full time allotted will be very effective.

Sit at the receiver's right side facing the Hara. Work with whichever hand feels most natural and comfortable for you. Starting at the lower right quadrant near the ileocecal valve, apply gentle palm pressure in a clockwise circular fashion, pressing along the rib margins, the space between hip and ribs, and along the front of the pelvic structure. Work with the breathing, one press per exhalation (Figure 9).

10. Place the heels of both palms alongside the rectus abdominus muscle (the "washboard" muscle in the center of the abdomen), with your fingertips grasping the opposite edge of the rectus abdominus. Working your hands like a cat "making biscuits" gently push-pull up and down the length of rectus abdominus muscle for a couple of minutes. As you work you may be able to increase your depth of pressure. This is an excellent technique for massaging the intestinal area and should be used regularly for anyone with constipation and sluggish digestion (Figure 10).

11. Place one hand over the navel and make brisk, superficial circles in a clockwise direction, warming the navel and the area just below it (Dan Tien area). Keep your hand relaxed and soft for maximum contact. If you do this for several minutes, the client may begin to feel a deep comfortable warmth or strengthening effect in the abdomen. As the abdomen relaxes slow the pace and deepen the pressure (Figure 11).

Figure 9	Figure 10	Figure 11

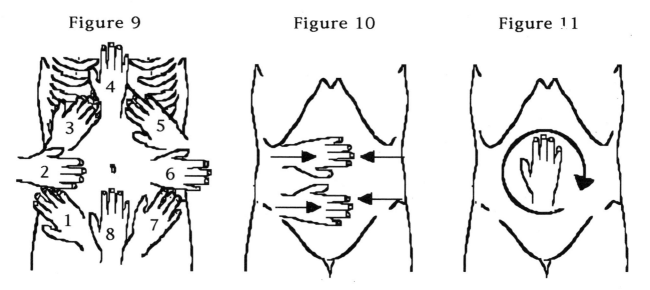

Treatment for the Legs and Feet

12. Next treat the front and sides of the legs with palm pressure down the Yang channels, from hip down to the feet. The Gall Bladder and Stomach Channels are in this area, and they frequently have sensitive points, so work carefully. Key points are ST-36, GB-34, GB-40 and GB-41 (Figure 12). Let your "mother hand" rest lightly on the Hara while working the leg channels. If this is comfortable for the receiver, you may apply thumb pressure to trace these channels.

Figure 12

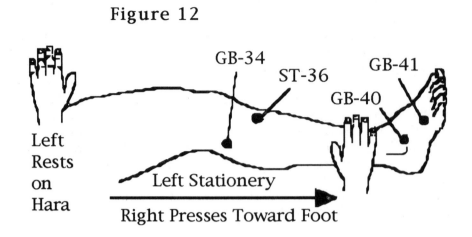

13. To treat the inner leg, start at the big toe joint, and use palm pressure to press upwards toward the hip area (Figure 13). The Spleen, Liver, and Kidney channels are in this area. Avoid the groin/genital area. The medial edge of the shin bone (tibia) (Spleen and Liver channels) is often quite tender with fibromyalgia. Key points in this section are SP-3, Ki-3, Liv-3 (the three source points), Ki-7, Sp-6, and Liv-8. Expect all to be sensitive. Just touching the points with light finger pressure for a few moments will help them to release.

Figure 13

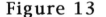

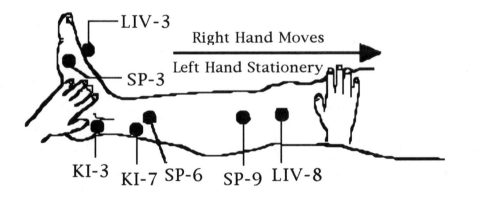

Foot massage: Sit at the client's feet; work with them one at a time. Use thumb pressure all over the sole of the foot to give thorough coverage. If you are familiar with the foot reflexology model, you may note where the most reactive areas are, and determmine which organ or body areas they are related to.

Press all around the calcaneus (heel bone) on both sides; there are good sleep-balancing reflex points located on both sides here. Grasp the joint where the large toe joins the foot, and with your other hand, grasp the joint where the smallest toe joins the foot, and work the foot like "scissors." This helps loosen up the connective tissue, fascia, and other structures between the metatarsals (bones of the foot), releasing tension in the body.

Then use one palm on the sole of the foot, one palm on top of the foot, and simply squeeze the whole foot firmly but gently between your hands. Finally, grasp the heel in one hand, and the toes in the other, and rotate the ankle joint 5-6 times in each direction. Repeat all steps for the other foot.

PART 2: BACK OF THE BODY

14.   Have the receiver turn to a face-down position and sit at her head. Place both hands on area between the scapulae (shoulder blades) in the upper back and administer alternating palm pressure in this area. Work rhythmically in a way that produces some upper body rocking as if you were "walking" your hands about on the person's upper back and shoulders (Figure 14). Many people with fibromyalgia have a great deal of discomfort and tension in this area; work at your partner's comfort level; strive for the "good hurt" comfort level.

15.   Use thumb pressure and work along the lower neck vertebrae. Press into the sides of the spinous processes; this is a good technique for releasing upper back and lower neck tension. You may work the section from approximately C-5 to T-8 in this manner (Figure 15).

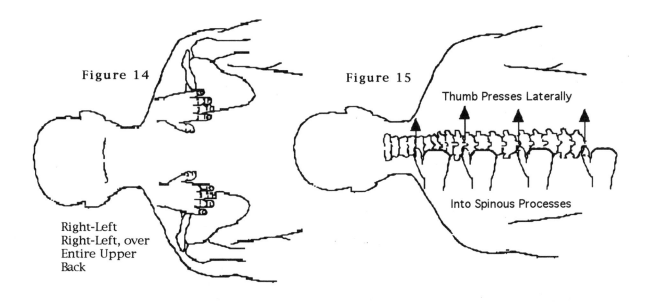

16.   Treat the entire Bladder meridian with palm pressure. Start at the shoulder blade area and work downward toward the hips and sacrum. You can work one side at a time by having one hand stationery (mother hand) on the upper back, and moving the other rhythmically giving palm pressure all the way to the sacrum (Figure 16). Work with the breathing pattern of the client. Treat both sides, making at least three repetitions down the back on each side.

If palm pressure is well received, you can then give thumb pressure, giving attention to both the Bladder lines on each side of the spine. (Appendix 5). The Bladder channel separates into two pairs of lines on the back; the inner pair of lines contains the Back-Shu points or Yu points which balance the internal functions, and the outer pair of lines relate to the emotional expressions of the various organs.

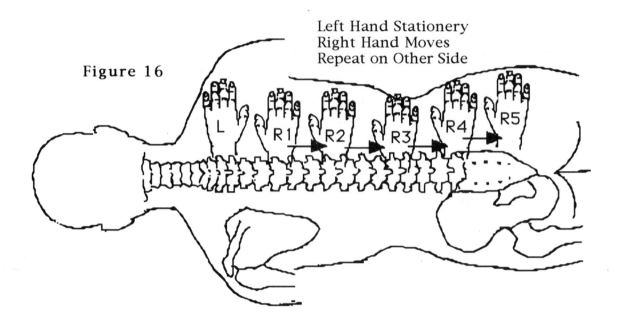

Figure 16

Left Hand Stationery
Right Hand Moves
Repeat on Other Side

17. When doing floor-work shiatsu, you may prefer to treat both sides of the back simultaneously (Figure 17).

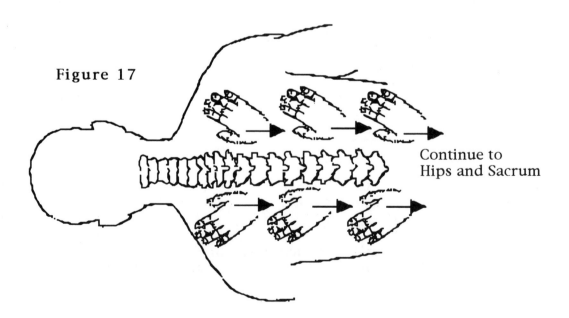

Figure 17

Continue to
Hips and Sacrum

18. Integrate the back by doing diagonal stretching: right hip and left shoulder, then left hip and right shoulder (Figure 18); repeat 4-6 times. Hold each stretch for 1 or 2 breaths. Then place one hand over the low back or hips and gently rock the pelvis back and forth for 30-60 seconds.

Figure 18   Diagonal Stretches

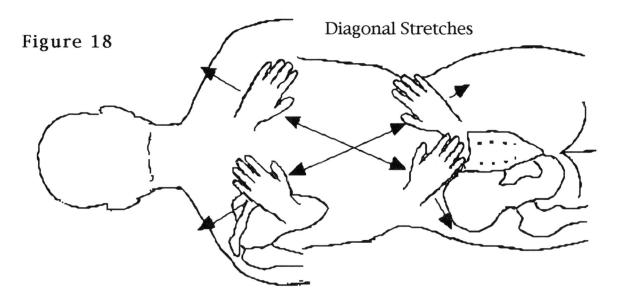

19. Next work with the hips and sacrum. Use gentle palm pressure to outline the triangular shape of the sacrum (Figure 19). There is frequently sacro-iliac joint pain with fibromyalgia, so work carefully. When you find particularly sensitive "spots" hold a little pressure there for 30-60 seconds, until you feel a pulsing sensation or other signal that release has occurred. Press on the sacrum itself, using palm pressure or thumb pressure to give thorough coverage. The sacrum area will probably be puffy and tender. Apply a circular palm stroke all over the sacrum and sacro-iliac joint area; rub briskly to generate some movement in the area and a feeling of warmth in the sacrum and low back. Next treat the gluteal muscles by starting at the posterior superior iliac spine (PSIS), and working laterally across the iliac crest. Use thumb pressure if possible; if too intense, switch to palm pressure.

20. Follow the contour of the pelvic crest from the center around to the hip joint itself, and then work all around the greater trochanter, holding points which are tight or tender (Figure 20). Repeat this line of points 2-3 times. Then work the fleshy part of the buttocks with palm pressure. The sciatic nerve travels beneath the gluteals, and is often pressure-sensitive. You are working with the Bladder channel and the Gall Bladder channel in the hip area.

Figure 19   **Figure 20**

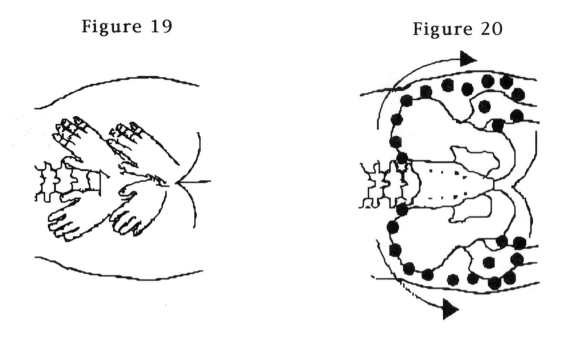

21. Work the back of the legs next. Place one hand on the sacrum (mother hand) and press along the Bladder channel from the top of the hamstrings all the way to the Achilles tendon (Figure 21). Use only (very) pressure on the back of the knee joint because there are nerves and vessels there which can be injured. Repeat 2-3 times to give good coverage of the hamstrings and calf muscles. If possible, change to thumb pressure and trace the meridians again once or twice.

Figure 21

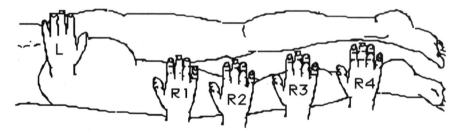

22. Closing and integrative movements: Briskly brush down the entire Bladder meridian from shoulders to heels with your palms. Also brush down the outside of the legs (Gall Bladder) and even down the arms from shoulder to hand. As a final technique, stand or sit at receiver's left side, and place your right hand middle finger lightly at the bottom of the sacrum (Du-2). With your left hand, middle finger, touch the lumbo-sacral joint. Hold this connection for 3-4 breaths. Then, with each breath the client takes, slide your left finger up one vertebra, and lightly touch the tip of the spinous process. Your two contact points will be getting further apart with each breath. Continue up the back of the neck and skull, ending at the crown of the head (Du-20) with the left hand. The right hand remains stationery throughout (Fig. 22).

This is a powerfully calming technique which activates the parasympathetic nervous system and assists the client to become extremely deeply relaxed. Hold the final pair (Du-2 and Du-20) for 30-60 seconds, and then slowly withdraw your left hand first, then the right hand, when its time to break contact. Thank your client for the privilege of working with her. Make sure your client arises slowly, and make sure the balance and equilibrium is fine before they stand. Getting up too quickly can induce a bit of dizziness in some people. Give them a bit of time to wake up and be sure they are alert and centered if they need to drive or return to work after the session.

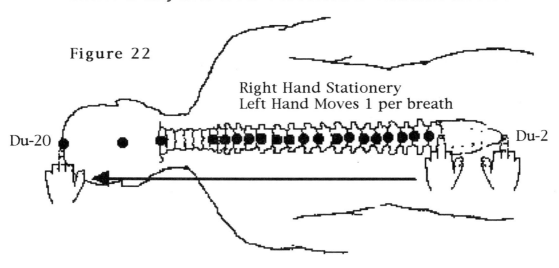

Figure 22

Right Hand Stationery
Left Hand Moves 1 per breath

Du-20   Du-2

MERIDIAN RELEASE TECHNIQUE

A further refinement of the general shiatsu routine is to spend some time working with one or more meridians which may be particularly stiff, painful or achy. First have the person show you where it hurts. They may color the areas on the blank body chart, or indicate by pointing to the areas. Then refer to the meridian charts in Appendix A and identify which meridians may be affected. The receiver may be able to help you select the best ones to work with by looking at the charts also. Have the nearby as you work (unless you are familiar enough with the meridians that you no longer need the charts).

Place one finger on the area the receiver has identified as most sensitive, and have them note the level of soreness or reactivity when you press lightly. You can ask them to use a subjective scale of 1 to 10, with 10 being the worst and 1 being non-reactive. As you work with other points on the same meridian, you can check from time to time as to the changes which are occurring. Also notice any particular sensations you can feel in the area, such as temperature, pulsing sensation, tissue texture, surface coloration, and so on.

Next, consult the chart for point locations, and select a point on the same meridian which is near the sensitive one. Touch it with a finger of your other hand. Notice if you can detect a pulsing sensation in either or both of the points. If you can, monitor the pulsing as you hold, until the

hold points until rhythm is same in both hands

rhythm and intensity is the same in both points. Still holding the original point with one hand, move your other hand and make contact with another point on the same meridian a bit further away from the original one. Hold both points and wait for the pulsing sensation in each to equalize. When they are equalized, move to the next point further away on the meridian, and repeat the procedure.

3-4 minutes may be needed to balance points

You may continue all the way to the end of the meridian, working point by point. Some points may release or equalize more quickly than others. It is not uncommon to hold a pair of points as much as three or four minutes in order to release tense tissues. This is slow, meditative work and the receiver will probably find it very relaxing and nurturing. When you reach the end of the meridian, check the target point again. The person may tell you that it feels much less painful. If the release is only slight, you may work points on the other side of the painful points, going toward the other end of the meridian. For example, if the shoulder is painful in the area of Large Intestine-15 and 16, you may first work down toward the hand, touching LI-14, LI-13, LI-11, LI-10, LI-8, LI-5, LI-4, LI-2. Then work the points on the Large Intestine meridian along its course into the neck and head.

After working the entire meridian, you may ask the person again for a new rating of the pain or reactivity. In most cases, it will be significantly better than when you started. If you did not attain much improvement, then check a different meridian in the same general area. For example, if the Large Intestine points gave only partial release, next you might try using Lung meridian points or Small Intestine points in combination with the original painful points.

Check "paired" meridians for more release

If you have studied Chinese medicine and are familiar with the paired relationships of the meridians this may help you select other meridians which will help. For example, when the Gall Bladder meridian is tight, using its paired meridian, the Liver, may be helpful. The anatomical relationships may also help if you are familiar with them. For example pain in the front of the thigh (Quadriceps muscles, Stomach meridian) may be helped by working points on the meridian in the back of the thigh (Hamstring muscles, Bladder meridian.) If you work with the same person on a regular basis, you can take one painful area at a time over a series of sessions, and identify the best release points for that person's aches and pains. You may also show them where to work. You may mark the points with magraine pellets or with a tiny dot of water-color ink, so they can find the points later on their own.

As people experience more and more bodywork, they can often become very good at feeling the "connections" between the various points. They can often distinguish which points seem to give the most relief also, thereby becoming a powerful enabler of their own therapeutic progress. When a person reaches this level of body awareness, they can participate much more effectively in the therapeutic partnership with their bodywork therapist or friend who is doing this work with them.

meridian release can be done alone or with Shiatsu

The meridian release procedure can be done in conjunction with the Shiatsu sequence or it can serve as a stand-alone mini-treatment.

Chapter 12

Client Education
for Health Empowerment

INTRODUCTION TO CLIENT EDUCATION

One of the greatest responsibilities of holistic health care practitioners is to educate and empower the client to do much more for himself. For those who have chronic conditions such as chronic fatigue and fibromyalgia, it is not a question of whether there is anything a person can do to get better, it is a question of where to start. While mainstream medicine is rather limited in what it has to offer the person with chronic illness, the holistic field has so much to offer that it can be overwhelming at first, especially when many modalities are unfamiliar and based on principles that seem strange to Western people. This chapter will present ideas for assisting the client to explore some of the numerous ways he/she can start to take better care of his/her own health.

When working with a client who is ready and willing to make lifestyle changes, it is important to start slowly and give the person support along the way. Who has not tried to make a change, such as starting an exercise program, eating healthier foods, or quitting smoking without failing numerous times? Many clients have a history of such experiences and don't have much confidence or self-esteem about these areas. Those with chronic fatigue or fibromyalgia may have limited capacity to make changes due to their pain, low energy, depression, or inability to concentrate or remember details. They may need a few sessions of acupuncture or bodywork and start to feel better before they can begin to entertain the idea of making fundamental lifestyle changes.

First find out if the client is interested AND WILLING to start making changes that will yield beneficial progress in her health. Some clients will want to start right away; others are still waiting for someone or something to "cure them." If she says no, do not be offended, do not nag, do not try to persuade, do not try to convince. This is only the first mentioning of the subject. In general, people have had enough of being told what to do, and even if they aren't ready to adopt any lifestyle changes, continuing to talk about the subject may create resistance or cause the client to leave therapy. This is not a win-win situation! Be patient with her; many times, when the person starts to feel better, she will start to get curious and motivated to do something for herself. Sometimes it will take a relapse or two. When she is ready and willing to begin making changes, spend a little time exploring the options. Some of the major categories for change are:

- Sleep improvement
- Nutrition (diet, supplements, green drinks, etc.)
- Movement (walking, stretching, Yoga, Qi Gong, etc.)
- Meditation/relaxation/imagery
- Self-exploration (counselling, 12-step progrrams, self-help books and tapes)
- Home therapies (aromatherapy, acupressure points, skin brushing)
- Stress management

Ask the client which categories interest her at the present time. She may be attracted to one or more, and repelled by others. Someone who has been on numerous diets and weight loss plans may be repelled by the idea of yet another attempt at what she has failed so many times. Be prepared with resources to help the person in each of these categories. Reading lists, local instructors who teach meditation or yoga, magazine articles, web sites can be shared with clients. Things you can teach them, such as acupoints to work, stretches, breathing and supplements are all excellent. Therapists can prepare take-home literature in each of the areas they frequently recommend to help clients get started.

The remainder of this chapter contains some of the client education materials I have developed over the years. The first is a health evaluation that the client takes. You may want to go through it with her, helping with interpretation of each item. Because it is based on the holistic paradigm, it will elevate self-awareness and help the person identify areas where core imbalances have been present. From those she can select areas that may have especially strong leverage for her.

The second item is the "Energy Management Strategy". This is a simple model to help the client can see how the many possible approaches fit into an energetic framework based on traditional Chinese medicine. She is encouraged to select items from each of the three categories: conserving the energy she still has, getting the energy moving, and rebuilding weak or deficient energy. I have had excellent feedback on this; clients say that it helps them understand the purpose of all the different modalities, and puts pieces of a puzzle together to form an integrated view of what they are trying to do. It also gives a structure for choosing modalities that work well together to achieve therapeutic outcomes.

The third item shows how to use self-massage or acupressure, illustrating several of the most commonly used acupoints and which symptoms they treat. Be sure to show the client how to work the points. Let them feel how much pressure to apply, how long to stimulate, and other factors which will help them with the "how to". This can also be used by family members or friends who would like to do something to help their loved one.

The fourth item is a one-page summary of many techniques that can be used for symptomatic relief of pain, depression, fatigue, and sleeplessness. It can help the client select the most effective approaches for her symptoms.

Next is an article which can be given to new clients. I ask them to read through it and think about what is says for the first week or two. Later I ask them what, if anything, in the article appealed to them for self-help. I have been pleasantly surprised at responses I have received. Some have said "I thought I'd tried just about everything, but now I realize there is much more", or "It gave me hope that I can get better," or "There are several things in there that I know I can start to do right away."

Next there is a section entitled "Twelve Easy Things", which was previously published in an earlier book called "Oriental Bodywork and Fibromyalgia Syndrome" (That book is no longer in print, having been replaced by the present volume). The final section is "Frequently Asked Questions" to help with some of the more common questions and concerns of those with fibromyalgia and chronic fatigue.

⑦ SIGNS OF HEALTH IN TRADITIONAL CHINESE MEDICINE: A FOCUS ON BEING

Almost everyone has taken a self-evaluation health quiz. They frequently appear in women's magazines, general health magazines, wellness profiles given by employers or HMO's, even the Sunday supplement. By taking the quiz and adding up the score, the individual can determine his stress levels and general condition of health. Usually there are about ten questions which evaluate the person's health related behaviors such as smoking, drinking, exercise, cholesterol, fat and salt intake, usage of a relaxation technique, and wearing seat belts. A person who avoids the unhealthy items and practices the healthy ones gets a high score and is deemed very healthy.

It is easy to get the feeling that something is missing in these health quizzes. Many people know someone who scored very high (maybe even themselves!) but they are miserably depressed, have some dangerous medical condition, or their life is a mess. On the other hand, there are people who flagrantly abuse these criteria, and yet they are productive, happy, have rich wonderful relationships, and seem to have less stress than many. These common health evaluations and most of the wellness and stress management programs in our hospitals, clinics, and fitness centers focus on behavioral aspects of life. In other words, they look at what we are "doing." Little, if any, emphasis is given to how we are "being" as a way of assessing health status.

The holistic medical traditions of the East, including traditional Chinese medicine have, for thousands of years, placed much greater importance on the "being" part of life. After all, the "doings" are just a means to an end which is often characterized as self-mastery, enlightenment, or spiritual awakening. This section offers a different set of criteria for assessing one's health. These are the "Seven Signs of Health in Traditional Chinese Medicine," and can be very valuable for staying on track and identifying imbalances long before they become actual sickness or pathology. They are weighted with different point values, with a total of 100 possible points. Use it along with the standard western evaluations, for health-related habits and behaviors ARE important, and people can create a much deeper understanding of their stress and health challenges in both "doing" AND "being."

SEVEN SIGNS OF HEALTH
IN TRADITIONAL CHINESE MEDICINE

1. <u>Physical and mental stamina and resilience; ability to follow through and complete tasks and projects; NO FATIGUE.</u> (Max. 5 points).

In health, a person has all the energy needed to do his life's work, to bounce back from disappointments, setbacks, and failures; and to set goals and take steps to achieve them. To be tired and ready for rest at the end of a full and productive day is normal and expected, but many people in our society suffer from continuous fatigue in varying degrees. For some it is mental fatigue and for others it is physical. Fatigue is the FIRST SIGN of an imbalance in Chinese Medicine because it indicates a depletion of the Qi, or vital energy of the person.

Depletion of Qi often comes from overwork (mental or physical), chronic worry or anxiety, inappropriate nourishment (physical or emotional), or not attending to our needs; the things we Westerners call "Stress."

2. <u>Good appetite for food, life, personal growth, change study, and learning</u> (Max. 5 points).

This item relates to the enthusiasm and enjoyment of "taking in", where the first one relates to our ability to "give out". Taken together, they represent a dynamic balance (Yin/Yang) of our interaction with other people, our work, environment, and the process of moving along through life. There are many people who are "stuck" at one spot in their personal growth, and fear, anger, grief, worry, or numbness prevent them from taking in life to the fullest.

3. <u>Good sleep; can fall asleep quickly and wake up refreshed, relaxed, and centered; dreams relate to future events and problem-solving.</u> (Max. 5 points)

Amount and quality of sleep are important indicators of the balance between Yin and Yang. Too much sleep or not enough sleep are both signs of disharmony. Dreams about the past reflect an imbalance that was manifest at that time. Sad, weird, or scary dreams indicate an illness condition. Dreams in which good ideas or insights or information come are excellent signs (..."an Angel of the Lord appeared in a dream"...sound familiar?). In Western medicine also, dreams and sleep quality are important indicators of health.

4. <u>Good Memory</u> (Max. 10 points).

In Chinese medical theory, all phenomena can be classified and subdivided into their Yin and Yang aspects. The Chinese recognize two types of memory. "Relative memory" relates to digital data and indicates a Yang condition. There are many people who can remember phone numbers, stock codes, names, prices, and so on; these are things we think of as digital, or "left brain" functions according to Western science. "Image memory" relates to visuals, feelings, melodies and other "right brain" functions, and indicates a more Yin condition. There are people who will say "I never forget a face, but the names escape me," or can match colors from memory, or remember a melody after one listening. Good memory of both types is an indication of healthy balance.

5. <u>Always cheerful and pleasant; never angry (anger is always our own fault), no grousing or complaining</u> (Max. 10 points).

It is not uncommon for some individuals to become irritated by this notion of accepting responsibility (response-ability) for our emotions, disposition, and attitudes. We Americans live in a society which teaches us to place the locus of control and blame outside of ourselves. The number of lawsuits which seek to assign blame to others (individuals, corporations, physicians, the government, the police, etc.) is extravagantly beyond the number of reasonable claims. When a person can move to a level of personal evolution where he accepts total responsibility for his choices, understand his emotional responses as communication from within about what he might need to change, and remain pleasant-tempered even under stressful conditions, h e has made a very large step toward healthful being.

6. <u>Easy decision-making; quick reflexes with no accidents. (Maximum 10 points).</u>

There are two considerations in this item. The first one, easy decision-making, depends on three factors. First, easy decision-making relates to clarity about what one wants. Second, the person must have good criteria for evaluating choices. Third, there must be good good feedback mechanisms to know if one is getting what he wants.   For some people decisions are a struggle in only a few contexts, such as buying decisions, or what they want to eat. For others, almost every decision is a source of struggle and stress. They usually end up being the puppets of someone who likes being in charge and controlling others, and who can make decisions easily.

The second part of this item, quick reflexes with no accidents, indicates one's ability to respond to and operate in the external environment. There are people that we call "accident-prone" who are always bumping into objects, falling down, slipping and other accidents. This suggests a problem in their ability to input and respond to sensory information or their inability to distinguish where they end and the outside world begins. For some people, the problem lies in their inability to focus attention and avoid distraction. I n health, with the sensory faculties sharp and the neurological circuits firing well, a person moves lightly and gracefully, in good harmony with other objects and beings in her/his proximity.

7. <u>Appreciation and gratitude; a sense of higher purpose and being part of something bigger; acknowledge problems as opportunities; never having to lie to oneself or others</u> (Max. 55 points.)

This is the big one; more than half the total points come from this item. Appreciation and gratitude are truly the mark of an evolved person. The ability to maintain inner peace even during stressful situations, is a high achievement. Chinese wisdom regards arrogance as the most serious of all possible illnesses because it shows that the person is out of touch with his place in the universal order of things. He has lost his sense of connection and oneness with all of life and with the spiritual world.

A sense of purpose which relates to some form of service, teaching or healing (in the broadest sense) is also a very positive state. Many people who have discovered their "calling" describe an immediate transformation which occurred and changed their lives from that point forward. In the same vein, the wise and mature individual knows that our problems and difficulties in life are the teachers we need in order to come to our wisdom and maturity; therefore each problem or obstacle is an opportunity to learn a new skill or discover a new facet of life, or develop an inner characteristic such as patience, forgiveness, or compassion.

Never having to lie to self or others is a concept which is well known by the millions of people who have attained sobriety through the Twelve Steps of Alcoholics Anonymous. The fourth step in the twelve-step recovery process entails "making a fearless and searching moral inventory of ourselves." We must learn to recognize and acknowledge our strengths and gifts as well as our weaknesses and challenges. To make the most significant and lasting positive changes in one's health and well-being, it is important to identify the tell tale signs of the imbalances that are there, and what needs to be done to learn to rebuild the internal harmony of health.

This evaluation is quite different than the one where you score high if you don't smoke, don't drink over "X" alcoholic drinks per week, exercise a couple times a week, watch your cholesterol, fat and salt intake, practice a relaxation technique, and don't have casual sex with strangers. Certainly those health-promoting behaviors are important, but our lives and our selves are much more than just a collection of habits, behaviors, and medical diagnostic report sheets. We are human "beings", so how we are "being" is greater than the sum of all the "doings" we are doing.

[handwritten margin notes at top: Chinese medicine — all dis-ease and illness arises from the imbalances of Vital Substances: qi - blood - Essence and Shen]

ENERGY MANAGEMENT STRATEGY

Individuals who are recovering from chronic illness can begin to organize their lifestyle choices around the concept of learning to manage their energy more effectively. From the point of view of Chinese medicine, all dis-ease and illness arises from imbalances of the Vital Substances: Qi, Blood, Essence, and Shen. When Qi becomes deficient, amounts are insufficient to support all the functions of Qi, including warming, transforming, protecting, moving, and retaining organs and substances in their places. If Blood becomes deficient, there is impairment of its functions including moistening, nourishing, maintaining, and regulating cyclical activities. Qi and Blood can also become stagnant or blocked so that its flow is choppy, irregular, uneven, or unpredictable, resulting in pain symptoms.

There are three parts to this energy management strategy. First the individual must take measures to conserve the energy she/he still has. The individual has probably gotten into a health crisis because of choices which have allowed her energy to become depleted over time. The first step is to "stop the leaks". This will entail evaluation of the individual's stress patterns, and making changes which will allow her to conserve energy. *[handwritten: ① stop the energy leaks]*

The second part is to begin to rebuild the body's energy. Regenerating the immune system, strengthening the Organs which produce, store, and govern the energy, and rebuilding blood quality are the key components of this part. *[handwritten: ② rebuild body's energy]*

The third part of the strategy is to stimulate the movement of Qi and Blood. Stagnation patterns usually accompany deficiency patterns, and the pain and discomfort of fibromyalgia are a result of stagnation. Restoring movement helps reduce pain, relieves depression and anxiety, and helps many digestive symptoms. *[handwritten: ③ stimulate the movement of qi + blood]*

The illustration on the next page summarizes the energy management strategy. There are three circles for the three parts of the process: conserving, rebuilding, and moving energy. Each circle contains a list of methods, modalities, and strategies which facilitatie that aspect of energy management.

The client can select something new from each of the three circles to start her energy management strategy. Encourage her to select something that would be simple and easy, so she can experience success right away. After two or three weeks, she can add something else from each category if appropriate. I recommend that people educate themselves about the techniques they think they would like to use. Some things take quite a bit of time, energy, money, or space. Others are as simple as taking a supplement every day. Some have the potential to ignite a lifelong journey, others can fit right in to their present lifestyle.

<u>Strategies for Recovery</u>
Fibromyalgia and Chronic Fatigue Syndrome

Energy Management Strategy

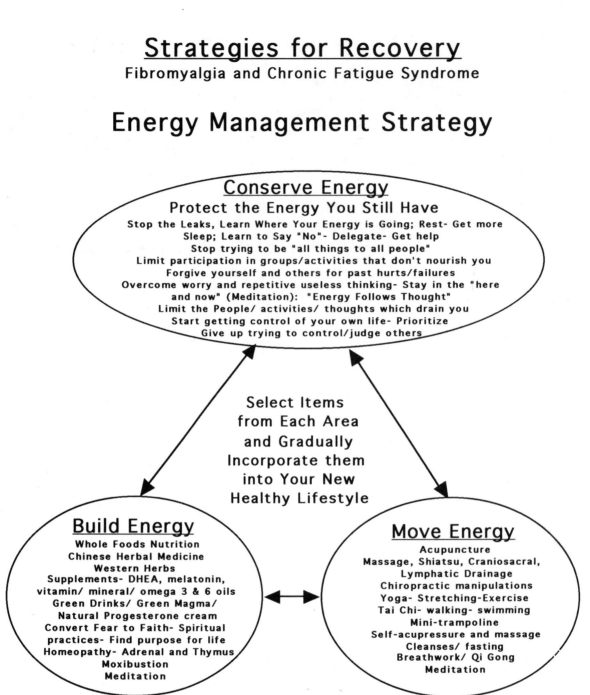

<u>Conserve Energy</u>
Protect the Energy You Still Have
Stop the Leaks, Learn Where Your Energy is Going; Rest- Get more
Sleep; Learn to Say "No"- Delegate- Get help
Stop trying to be "all things to all people"
Limit participation in groups/activities that don't nourish you
Forgive yourself and others for past hurts/failures
Overcome worry and repetitive useless thinking- Stay in the "here
and now" (Meditation): "Energy Follows Thought"
Limit the People/ activities/ thoughts which drain you
Start getting control of your own life- Prioritize
Give up trying to control/judge others

Select Items
from Each Area
and Gradually
Incorporate them
into Your New
Healthy Lifestyle

<u>Build Energy</u>
Whole Foods Nutrition
Chinese Herbal Medicine
Western Herbs
Supplements- DHEA, melatonin,
vitamin/ mineral/ omega 3 & 6 oils
Green Drinks/ Green Magma/
Natural Progesterone cream
Convert Fear to Faith- Spiritual
practices- Find purpose for life
Homeopathy- Adrenal and Thymus
Moxibustion
Meditation

<u>Move Energy</u>
Acupuncture
Massage, Shiatsu, Craniosacral,
Lymphatic Drainage
Chiropractic manipulations
Yoga- Stretching-Exercise
Tai Chi- walking- swimming
Mini-trampoline
Self-acupressure and massage
Cleanses/ fasting
Breathwork/ Qi Gong
Meditation

Self Acupressure For Fibromyalgia and Chronic Fatigue

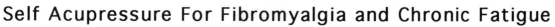

Find the point or area which helps the symptom.
Apply firm pressure or massage to the point or
area for one to two minutes.

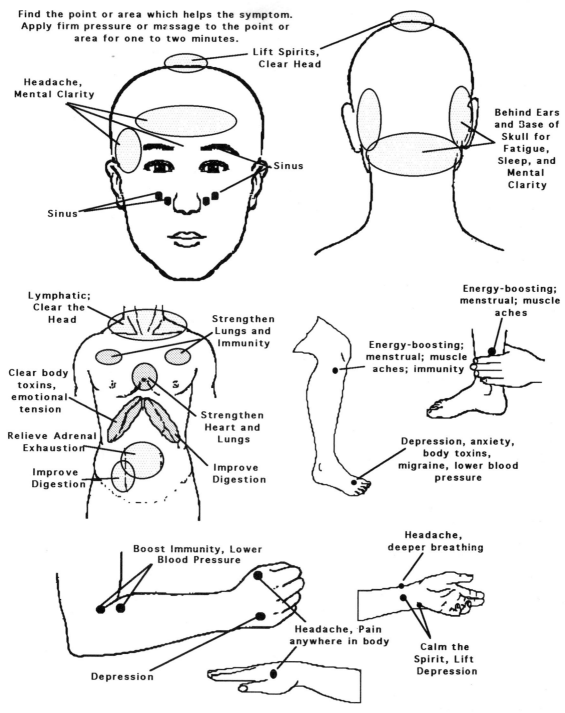

Lift Spirits, Clear Head

Headache, Mental Clarity

Sinus

Sinus

Behind Ears and Base of Skull for Fatigue, Sleep, and Mental Clarity

Lymphatic; Clear the Head

Strengthen Lungs and Immunity

Clear body toxins, emotional tension

Strengthen Heart and Lungs

Relieve Adrenal Exhaustion

Improve Digestion

Improve Digestion

Energy-boosting; menstrual; muscle aches

Energy-boosting; menstrual; muscle aches; immunity

Depression, anxiety, body toxins, migraine, lower blood pressure

Boost Immunity, Lower Blood Pressure

Headache, deeper breathing

Headache, Pain anywhere in body

Depression

Calm the Spirit, Lift Depression

SELF HELP AND NATURAL THERAPY FOR
FIBROMYALGIA AND CHRONIC FATIGUE RECOVERY
It's Up to You!

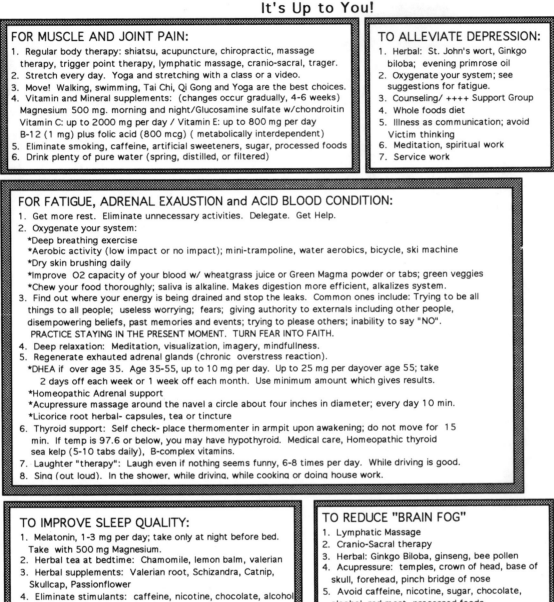

FOR MUSCLE AND JOINT PAIN:

1. Regular body therapy: shiatsu, acupuncture, chiropractic, massage therapy, trigger point therapy, lymphatic massage, cranio-sacral, trager.
2. Stretch every day. Yoga and stretching with a class or a video.
3. Move! Walking, swimming, Tai Chi, Qi Gong and Yoga are the best choices.
4. Vitamin and Mineral supplements: (changes occur gradually, 4-6 weeks)
   Magnesium 500 mg. morning and night/Glucosamine sulfate w/chondroitin
   Vitamin C: up to 2000 mg per day / Vitamin E: up to 800 mg per day
   B-12 (1 mg) plus folic acid (800 mcg) (metabolically interdependent)
5. Eliminate smoking, caffeine, artificial sweeteners, sugar, processed foods
6. Drink plenty of pure water (spring, distilled, or filtered)

TO ALLEVIATE DEPRESSION:

1. Herbal: St. John's wort, Ginkgo biloba; evening primrose oil
2. Oxygenate your system; see suggestions for fatigue.
3. Counseling/ ++++ Support Group
4. Whole foods diet
5. Illness as communication; avoid Victim thinking
6. Meditation, spiritual work
7. Service work

FOR FATIGUE, ADRENAL EXAUSTION and ACID BLOOD CONDITION:

1. Get more rest. Eliminate unnecessary activities. Delegate. Get Help.
2. Oxygenate your system:
   *Deep breathing exercise
   *Aerobic activity (low impact or no impact); mini-trampoline, water aerobics, bicycle, ski machine
   *Dry skin brushing daily
   *Improve O2 capacity of your blood w/ wheatgrass juice or Green Magma powder or tabs; green veggies
   *Chew your food thoroughly; saliva is alkaline. Makes digestion more efficient, alkalizes system.
3. Find out where your energy is being drained and stop the leaks. Common ones include: Trying to be all things to all people; useless worrying; fears; giving authority to externals including other people, disempowering beliefs, past memories and events; trying to please others; inability to say "NO".
   PRACTICE STAYING IN THE PRESENT MOMENT. TURN FEAR INTO FAITH.
4. Deep relaxation: Meditation, visualization, imagery, mindfullness.
5. Regenerate exhauted adrenal glands (chronic overstress reaction).
   *DHEA if over age 35. Age 35-55, up to 10 mg per day. Up to 25 mg per day over age 55; take
      2 days off each week or 1 week off each month. Use minimum amount which gives results.
   *Homeopathic Adrenal support
   *Acupressure massage around the navel a circle about four inches in diameter; every day 10 min.
   *Licorice root herbal- capsules, tea or tincture
6. Thyroid support: Self check- place thermomenter in armpit upon awakening; do not move for 15 min. If temp is 97.6 or below, you may have hypothyroid. Medical care, Homeopathic thyroid sea kelp (5-10 tabs daily), B-complex vitamins.
7. Laughter "therapy": Laugh even if nothing seems funny, 6-8 times per day. While driving is good.
8. Sing (out loud). In the shower, while driving, while cooking or doing house work.

TO IMPROVE SLEEP QUALITY:

1. Melatonin, 1-3 mg per day; take only at night before bed. Take with 500 mg Magnesium.
2. Herbal tea at bedtime: Chamomile, lemon balm, valerian
3. Herbal supplements: Valerian root, Schizandra, Catnip, Skullcap, Passionflower
4. Eliminate stimulants: caffeine, nicotine, chocolate, alcohol overstimulating activities in evening.
5. Self massage with sesame oil 1-2 hours before bedtime
6. Make a list of everything you need to do or remember the next day; empty your mind of busy thoughts.
7. Acupressure: inner ankles, inner wrists, temples, forehead, base of skull, abdomen.

TO REDUCE "BRAIN FOG"

1. Lymphatic Massage
2. Cranio-Sacral therapy
3. Herbal: Ginkgo Biloba, ginseng, bee pollen
4. Acupressure: temples, crown of head, base of skull, forehead, pinch bridge of nose
5. Avoid caffeine, nicotine, sugar, chocolate, alcohol, red meat, processed foods
6. Eliminate dairy and wheat for 1 month to test for allergy; also test others you suspect.
7. Dietary essent. oils: Omega 3 (fish oil) and Omega 6 (evening primrose or flaxseed oil)
8. B- Vitamins
9. Oxygenate the system (see under fatigue)

FIBROMYALGIA SYNDROME
CHRONIC FATIGUE SYNDROME
LIFESTYLE AND NUTRITION-BASED RECOVERY

It is quite feasible for people with fibromyalgia and chronic fatigue to regenerate their health to a high degree, or even to be healthier and more energetic than many of the people who have never had either of these illnesses! It is totally up to you- no one else can do it for you. Many suggestions given in this article are simple in concept but much more difficult to practice. The more of the items you do faithfully, the more fully you can come back from fibromyalgia or chronic fatigue to become the vibrant and dynamic person you were born to be. You may have to do numerous things which each contribute to your recovery. You may not begin to see substantial progress for two to four months, but stick with it anyway. Eventually, you may even be healthier than before you got sick. Getting better requires diligence, perseverance, commitment, time and money. It does not replace medical advice, and, if you want to, you should continue consulting with your medical doctor while working with the ideas presented here. You may not yet be ready for many of the items given here. If that is the case, do the things you can. If you only do one item, you will be helping your body get better.

1. Adopt A Spiritual Attitude Toward Your Health

Most people who encounter chronic illness spend large amounts of time and money looking for a wonder pill or a doctor that can fix their problems, or hoping that research will discover a new "magic bullet" for their illness. Most go through a phase of asking "Why me? What did I do to deserve this?" It is time to stop asking that question and take the point of view that your fibromyalgia or chronic fatigue is a "Wake-Up Call" to take control of your life, take a good hard look at how you are using your personal resources of time, energy, thought, and emotional investment, and make the decision to do whatever it takes to get well. Realize that no one can do it for you. Also realize that the process of taking charge and doing the things described here will transform your life in a positive way. You are not a helpless victim and you have the opportunity of a lifetime hidden within your illness. You can no longer regard your health program as an inconvenient annoyance which must be endured. Enter it with joy, positive expectations, a sense of curiosity and adventure. Illness is a transformational experience for you and everyone around you.

Recommended reading

Creating Health, by Deepak Chopra MD
Love, Medicine and Miracles, by Bernie S. Siegel, MD
Peace, Love, and Healing, by Bernie S. Siegel, MD
Spontaneous Healing, By Andrew Weill, MD
Full Catastrophe Living, by Jon-Kabat Zen

2. Find Out Where Your Energy Is Going and Recall It

Begin to become aware of all the people and activities in which you are investing your energy. You are probably also investing your energy in expectations, beliefs, rules, traditions, and memories that do not serve your health. For some people this may be the hardest step, and it will probably take some time and soul-searching. Working with a counsellor in private or group therapy or joining a twelve-step program will help you identify many of these drains on your energy and learn to disconnect from them.

You must also make decisions about where to invest your energy instead, and if you want to get well, you must put YOU and YOUR HEALTH high on the list. These must take priority over all your fears (rejection, abandonment, failure, change, disappointing someone), your past wounds (physical, emotional, psychological), old grudges or "scores" you have not settled, your expectations of perfection and being a super-human. You must disconnect from your past failures, guilt, sins, relationships, anger, and grief. End your affiliation with groups or individuals that take more of your energy than you can afford to give, and especially from those who take your energy without your consent. Over your lifetime you have established many "energy-links" with people and situations which you are now free to change. Start with the past: anything from the past that brings up negative feelings is something that is draining your energy all the time. If there are people in your life who drag you down or with whom you have emotionally draining interactions, you will want to sever those ties where you can, and learn better coping skills for dealing with spouse, parents, children, or others who are going to stay in your life. One by one, as you make final closure with the memories, events, people and beliefs that take your energy, you will be amazed at how much healthier and energetic you will become.

Recommended Reading

Anatomy of the Spirit, by Caroline Myss, Ph.D.
Living with Joy, by Sanaya Roman
Your Body Believes Every Word You Say, by Barbara Hoberman Levine
What You Feel, You Can Heal, by John Gray, Ph.D.
You Can Heal Your Life, by Louise Hay
The Dance of Anger, by Harriet Goldhor Lerner, Ph.D.
Bradshaw on The Family, by John Bradshaw (and others by
        Bradshaw)

---

3. Exercise

You must begin to move your body in a systematic, health-promoting manner every single day. The best exercises for recovering from fibromyalgia or chronic fatigue are walking, swimming, Yoga, Tai Chi, or Qi Gong. Walking is free. Swimming is excellent, though you may have to join a health club or YMCA to get year-round access to a pool, but you may also be able to join a yoga class or specialized water aerobics class at the same place (regular aerobics, even low-impact, is not appropriate for someone with severe fibromyalgia or chronic fatigue. Wait until you have more energy and strength). You can probably find a video on Tai Chi or Yoga in most video stores.

Start gradually, even if five minutes is all you can do at first. Initially, you will probably dislike doing this, and you may think your body feels worse when you exercise, but that is an illusion. Exercise helps your body return to normal functioning, and just like overcoming an addiction, there is an initial period of readjustment and "withdrawal" symptoms. Your body has been accumulating toxins and metabolic waste products such as lactic acid, which must be eliminated gradually, and this can feel unpleasant in the early stages. Work through this and gradually increase your time, and be careful not to over-exercise. Many people with fibromyalgia say that stretching does more to relieve their muscle pain and fatigue than any other thing they do.

Another extremely valuable physical activity is jumping on a trampoline. You can use a mini-trampoline at home two to ten minutes per day to activate the lymphatic system, which is part of the immune system. Sluggish lymphatic system is a characteristic of fibromyalgia, and getting the lymph moving will help with your energy level and your muscle and joint pain. Another benefit is that bouncing will get you breathing, which will oxygenate your blood, which will help reduce fatigue, foggy-headedness, and pain. Mini trampolines are inexpensive and are available at many stores that carry sporting goods. They can also be found frequently at yard sales and thrift stores for a small amount. People who have degenerative arthritis or spinal disk disease should not use a trampoline. Select a form of exercise which does not stress the joints excessively, such as swimming or walking.

Another excellent method to stimulate the lymphatic system is dry skin brushing. If your skin is very painful, start with a dry wash cloth and scrub yourself all over very briskly. It should only take two or three minutes to treat the whole body. Do this every day when you get up in the morning, after work, or at a time of day when your energy drops. After a couple of weeks, shift to a brush made of natural vegetable fiber or loofa. Do not use synthetic fiber or animal hair brushes for skin brushing! You can purchase a vegetable fiber brush or loofa in any supermarket or shop which carries skin-care or massage supplies.

Recommended Reading

Stretching, by Bob Anderson
Yoga: 28 Day Exercise Plan, by Richard Hittleman

---

4.   Daily Sunlight Exposure

Get at least thirty minutes of exposure to natural sunlight daily. Combine with #3 above, and get your sunlight while walking outside. No sunglasses! For the first thirty minutes let the sunlight enter your eyes, where it stimulates receptors in the brain. This helps alleviate fatigue, depression, and other symptoms. It also helps regulate cycles such as sleeping. For days when you cannot go outside, or when the sun is hidden by clouds, purchase full-spectrum light bulbs and put them in areas where you spend time. You can purchase full-spectrum bulbs for your regular lamps, or you can get full-spectrum tubes for your fluorescent fixtures. Lighting stores and health food stores often carry full-spectrum bulbs. They cost more than regular bulbs, but they are worth it! Regular fluorescent tubes contribute to fatigue, headache, and other symptoms. If you have them where you work, consider getting full-spectrum tubes for your work area even if you have to pay for them yourself. Get up at or before dawn to "catch the wave" of rising energy of the day. This may be difficult at first, but synchronizing your daily rhythm with the sun will help your body find a much better rhythm. Go to bed so that you can be fast asleep before 11 PM. This will facilitate the liver's nightly de-toxification activities and harmonize your biorhythm with the natural day/night cycles.

Recommended Reading

Light: Medicine of the Future, by Jacob Liberman, OD, Ph.D.

---

5. Start On A Program Of Regular Body Therapy

Oriental bodywork, acupuncture, chiropractic, craniosacral therapy, massage therapy, trigger point therapy, neuromuscular therapy, and physical therapy are all good choices. Regularity is important. I recommend one session per week in the beginning. A massage or bodywork session usually lasts one hour. You may later adopt a maintenance schedule of once per month. Find a therapist with experience working with fibromyalgia or chronic fatigue. It is essential to have a therapist you feel comfortable with and whose work is effective for you. Give a new therapist three or four sessions before you decide to if he/she is the one for you. Bodywork is an art and a science, and two people who practice the same modality will not necessarily have equal effectiveness for you.

Bodywork has many benefits. It will loosen tight and painful muscles and attachments, facilitate the flow of blood, (which means more oxygen and nutrients to your tissues); it assists the body in releasing and discharging toxins and metabolic waste products; it teaches you body awareness; it moves and balances the Qi (vital life force); it calms the nervous system and promotes good sleep; it balances the endocrine and immune functioning; it fills a basic human need for positive touch and unqualified positive regard.

Sensitivity to pressure is often part of fibromyalgia, so it is YOUR responsibility to communicate with your therapist about your comfort. You may find the work a bit uncomfortable at first and you may be sore the next day. This soreness is the same as when you start a new exercise program, and the next day you realize you have muscles you had forgotten about. Your muscles and organs have a chance to release built up toxins and waste products. You will work through this, and after a few sessions that reaction will subside as your body becomes accustomed to the work. Your therapist can give you suggestions to minimize the soreness after your session. Just like cleaning out a long-neglected closet, sometimes it gets worse before it gets better!!

Recommended Reading

Acupressure's Potent Points, by Michael Reed Gach
All mainstream bookstores have a good selection of books on massage
    and acupuressure.

---

6. Become Informed

By now you have noticed that there is a list of references after eacn section. The ones listed are readily accessible through local bookstores and libraries or on-line bookstores. Books, videos, audio-cassettes and information you can access through the internet are your link to the methods, ideas and attitudes of healing. You need to study and read about your illness from the medical perspective as well as from alternative/holistic point of view. If you take medications (prescription or over-the-counter), look them up in the Physician's Desk Reference at the library and read about the side effects and other information given, or ask your pharmacist or physician about potential side effects, including any new symptoms which have developed while you were using a medication.

Knowledge and information are what you will base your decisions and strategies upon. Act as though you are going to get a Ph.D. (Personal Health Doctorate) in this field. Plan regular time for reading, watching videos, and listening to cassettes. If you don't have a computer, virtually all college and university libraries now have internet access, as do many public libraries. They have people on staff who can help you get started You will be utterly amazed at the wealth of information you can access on the internet about fibromyalgia and chronic fatigue.

Recommended Audiocassette Programs On Healing

Magical Mind, Magical Body, by Deepak Chopra MD
Energy Anatomy, by Caroline Myss
Chronic Fatigue, by Deepak Chopra MD
Unconditional Life, by Deepak Chopra, MD
Ageless Body, Timeless Mind, by Deepak Chopra, MD
Peace, Love, and Healing, by Bernie S. Siegel, MD
Your Sacred Self, by Wayne Dyer

Other Recommended Sources Of Information

From Fatigued to Fantastic, Jacob Teitelbaum MD   Order from author at
    Deva Press, 139 Old Solomons Island Road, Annapolis MD 21401
Fibromyalgia and Chronic Myofascial Pain Syndrome: Survival Manual,
    by Devin Starlanyl and Mary Ellen Copeland
Reversing Fibromyalgia, by Dr. Joe M. Elrod

7. BEGIN TO RELEASE YOURSELF FROM DEPENDENCY ON DRUGS AND MEDICATIONS

Most medications are used to suppress symptoms. A few actually cure things (antibiotics), and some are necessary for certain illnesses or if you have had something removed (insulin for diabetics, thyroxin for someone who has had the thyroid gland removed). A few prevent short-term crisis (asthma inhalers). Here are some types of medications to strive to eliminate if you are taking: antidepressants, sleeping pills, pain killers, muscle relaxants, anti-inflammatory, antacids, steroids, synthetic hormone replacement, etc.

If you have over-the counter remedies or a prescription that you only use "as needed", such as for headaches, these you can stop yourself when you have used up the refills, or even before. Maintenance drugs that you take every day, such as antidepressants, should be reduced or eliminated only with the knowledge and co-operation of your medical doctor. Talk to the doctor about your goal to become as drug-free as you can. If the doctor seems to discourage you in this goal, consider changing doctors. You can learn to overcome most symptoms without drugs by restoring balance through natural alternatives. Many naturopathic physicians (ND's) and osteopathic physicians (DO) will work with you to get your body as free of chemicals as you can. They can prescribe medication when necessary, but also work with natural methods. More and more MD's are becoming aware of the importance of cutting down or eliminating drugs that are not absolutely necessary.

It is important for you to know that you have the right to full disclosure of all side-effects or dangers of any drug or procedure, and you have the right to refuse any diagnostic test or therapeutic intervention which is suggested. All drugs have side effects. Read the circular that comes with any medication (including over-the-counter products) and talk to your pharmacist or physician for any additional information you need. There are also on-line resources for learning about any pharmaceuticals you may be taking.

You cannot be fully vital and reach your full health potential if you are taking drugs to control symptoms. The short term benefits do not outweigh the long term side-effects and potential damage. If you have chronic fatigue or fibromyalgia and no other serious medical conditions (such as diabetes or heart disease), strive to become drug-free. According to Dr. Julian Whitaker, MD, Medical Editor for "Health and Healing", in 1996 160,000 Americans died from adverse reactions to prescription drugs. Eighteen million more suffered toxic side effects. Patients should carefully question their physicians and pharmacists about the appropriateness of drugs for their situation and consider natural alternatives when available.

Recommended Reading

The Menopause Years: the Wise Woman Way, by Susun Weed
Healthy Healing, by Linda Rector-Page, ND., Ph.D.
Reclaiming Your Health: Exploding the Medical Myth, by John Robbins

8. CLEAN UP YOUR DIET

You create your health every day by what you put into your body. This means not only your physical body, but the health of your mind, emotional processes, and ability to create spiritual connection. Most people who experience chronic fatigue and other chronic symptoms are routinely eating substances which are processed, chemicalized, refined and adulterated. You must eat natural foods if you want to optimize your health. Eliminate caffeine, alcohol, tobacco, hydrogenated oils and margarine, artificial sweeteners, refined sugar and flour, and dairy products first. Cut down on red meat, butter, eggs, and eliminate fried foods. Eat whole grains, vegetables, beans, and a small amount of fruit, with filtered or spring water. Eat fresh fish, organic chicken, or turkey for protein. A side-benefit will be shedding extra pounds you've been carrying around for years. You will need to use your will power, but it will get easier as you go along. If you have been eating any of the forbidden items above, especially caffeine and refined sugar, you may have developed addictions to them, and there will be a period of withdrawal as you start the process of releasing your body from these substances.

Be willing to seem a bit weird to people who are still eating the way you used to. If you have salad and brown rice for breakfast, that can become part of your new eccentric personality and soon you will become a role model for others who are suffering from chronic symptoms. There are dozens of excellent whole-foods cookbooks, and you may be able to find a class in macrobiotic or whole-foods cooking in your area. Check with health food stores and massage/bodywork schools for someone who can help. Many people have been told that their depression is due to a chemical imbalance and it takes drugs to correct the imbalance. It is true that someone who is depressed has a chemical imbalance and it is also true that you create your body chemistry every single day by what you eat and drink, your thoughts and activities. Do not buy into the myth; the vast majority of people (except those with bipolar disorder and other extreme psychotic illnesses) can change their body chemistry naturally with appropriate nutrition, exercise, and positive attitudes and thoughts. Work with your physician if you are taking maintenance medications.

Recommended Reading

Staying Healthy With the Seasons, by Elson Haas, MD
Food and Healing, by Annemarie Colbin
Healing with Whole Foods, by Paul Pitchford

---

9. Use Essential Oils (Aromatherapy), Supplements And Herbs To Help The Body Detoxify And Restore Itself

You may decide to go to a Chinese herbal practitioner; this can be extremely useful and effective for balancing many conditions including fibromyalgia and chronic fatigue. As with other practitioners, make sure the person you work with is well-trained and has extensive experience with your particular problem.

Whether you use Chinese herbal formulas or not, you will want to add a number of valuable nutritional supplements to your diet. Buy your supplements from a reputable health food store, mail order company, or at a grocery store which has a good selection of supplements. Do not be hypnotized by promises of miraculous cures from magic formulas or rare imported plants or other substances. Botanicals will probably have a place in your recovery program, but it will not be one isolated product that will reverse your illness. Only add one or two things at a time, and use a new product for a minimum of six weeks before deciding if it is helping.

The five major areas for supplements suggested are A) Oils B) Vitamins and minerals C) Anti-oxidants D) Western herbs and E) other natural products. You can find excellent reference material on supplements at the end of this section. I encourage you to read and learn about each item as you incorporate it into your diet. Taking supplements "consciously", that is, understanding what they do and how they benefit your health enhances their effectiveness.

A) Dietary Oils (Essential Fatty Acids)

1) OMEGA-3 is eicosapentanoic acid (EPA) and docosahexanoic acid (DHA). This can be obtained from FISH OIL (linolenic or omega 3 fatty acid)- Salmon oil is excellent for essential fatty acids. TAKE 1000 MG. PER DAY. Eat cold-water fish such as salmon, herring, mackerel, sardines twice or more per week.
2) OMEGA-6 is linoleic acid. Sources include evening primrose oil, sunflower oil (70%), and corn oil. (50%). Flaxseed oil has both omega-3 and omega-6 in proper balance. Boosts immune system. Take 1500 mg flaxseed oil or Evening Primrose Oil daily. The ideal balance is approximately 2:1 in favor of Omega-3.

These two dietary oils are essential for health of heart and vessels, cell walls, hormone production, rebuilding the immune system, nerve functioning, reducing inflammation, and some say protection against cancer. They can also reduce cholesterol.

B) Vitamins and Minerals

Take a good multivitamin/mineral product daily. Read the label and make sure it says the product is all natural. In addition to the multi, you may also add
1. Vitamin B-12- take daily 2 tabs
2. Magnesium- 500 mg before bed to promote sleep; helps with night sweats and muscle pain.

C) Anti-oxidants

These substances clean up "free radicals" which are the break-down products of chemicals, drugs, and pollutants we take in. The body does not know how to eliminate these, and they are implicated in several forms of cancer and other illness. Anti-oxidants help the body convert free radicals into substances it can deal with effectively. Several of the important ones are also vitamins and occur abundantly in fresh fruits and vegetables, especially eaten raw. Effects are not short term; take for two to three months to evaluate. Select one to take in addition to your multi-vitamin.

<u>Vitamin E</u> - up to 800 mg per day; also helps protect the nervous system and many other benefits. May be in your multi-vitamin in sufficient quantity.

<u>Vitamin C</u> - 1000 or more mg. per day; promotes oxygen delivery to brain for clearer thinking and many other benefits. Usually not enough in multi-vitamin products.

<u>Pycnogenol</u> - (proanthocyanindins) is one of the most powerful antioxidant products; take 3 20 mg. tabs per day, spread out through the day.

<u>Grape Seed Extract</u> - is also a powerful antioxidant and is less expensive than pycnogenol. Pycnogenol and Grape Seed extract are 20 times better antioxidants than vitamin C.

<u>Coenzyme Q-10</u> - is especially valuable for heart health, take one 30 mg capsule a day, take in morning only. It is also very expensive; try less expensive antioxidants first unless you have heart disease.

D) Individual Herbs

Use these for their special effects as indicated; follow dosages on bottle

<u>Ginger</u> - immune regulator; helps ulcer, migraine, reduces nausea; ginger essential oil has potential anti-inflammatory and/or anti-rheumatic properties.

<u>Ginkgo</u> - a strong antioxidant; immune booster, good for asthma; relieves fuzzy-headedness

<u>Cranberry</u> - antibiotic properties; good for urinary tract infection

<u>Echinacea</u> - antibiotic properties, supports immune system

<u>Goldenseal</u> - antibiotic properties; good for Candida

<u>Slippery Elm</u> - for heartburn and stomach discomfort

<u>Mexican (Wild) Yam</u> - has precursors for DHEA and progesterone; for menopausal symptoms

<u>Astragalus root</u> - boosts immune system

<u>Garlic</u> - immune booster and more

<u>Ginseng</u> - warms the system and boosts energy

E) Other Natural Products

<u>Natural Progesterone cream</u> - This has numerous benefits, including protecting women from heart disease, rebuilding bone, and many others. Relieves hot flashes and other menopausal symptoms. Takes away the dilemmas of synthetic hormone replacement therapy, and has no harmful side effects. Recommended for women over age 40 even if not yet menopausal, and not just for fibromyalgia and chronic fatigue patients. Should not be used by women with hormonally mediated cancers such as breast cancer and ovarian cancer.

<u>DHEA</u> -   the master adrenal hormone (dehydroepiandrosterone) occurs naturally in the body and decreases with chronic illness. Read the book before starting. Use the lowest dosage which gives results. Should not be used by women with hormonally mediated cancers such as breast cancer and ovarian cancer.

<u>Barley greens -</u> in tabs or powder, adds chlorophyll to your diet. This helps increase the oxygen capacity of the blood, making the system more alkaline, and helps your energy levels and combat fatigue. Use 3 to 6 tabs daily with meals, or equivalent powder in a "green drink". Wheatgrass juice has the same effect, very good.

<u>Melatonin -</u> a substance which is produced in the brain in response to sunlight. Helps promote restful sleep, and a strong antioxidant,   and   much more. Take only at night; 3 mg. Read the book before deciding to use melatonin.

<u>Glucosamine sulfate with chondroitin -</u> for some, helps fibromyalgia pain considerably. Rebuilds cartilage and connective tissue. Take for 3-6 months. 4 times a day, then go to maintenance dose of 1 or 2 times a day.

F) Aromatherapy

Aromatherapy is the use of essential oils of various plant species. They are applied to the skin in a massage oil blend or inhaled by diffusing in the home or work area. Aromatherapy is widely used in European hospitals, clinics, and homes because of its effectiveness and ease of usage. Essential oils add oxygen and nutrients to the body and help raise the vibrational energy (Qi or life force) for the person using them. They also gently assist the body to eliminate toxins and waste products from the cells and tissues. This is one of the most delightful and easy things you can do right away to improve your energy, comfort, mood and begin to cleanse your body. There are numerous books available in mainstream bookstores and information on the internet.

Recommended Reading

Staying Healthy With Nutrition, by Elson Haas, MD
Melatonin, the Anti-Ageing Hormone, by Suzanne LeVert
The DHEA Breakthrough, by Stephen Cherniske M.S.
What Your Doctor May not Tell You About Menopause, John Lee MD

10. Give Yourself a Soul-Nurturing Experience Every Day

This is an area where most modern people are sadly lacking. We have such busy, full lives but most of what we do drains us rather than replenishes us. A soul-nurturing experience is something you have total control over, that you can do any time, any place, any weather, that requires no other people, equipment, travel, etc. If you require other people to have your soul nourished, then you are dependent upon them and if they are not around or "don't feel like it", you have to go without. The ideal solution for a soul-nurturing experience is meditation. I strongly urge you to learn a meditation or relaxation exercise that you can do by yourself two or three times a day. Other examples include finding something beautiful in your surroundings, singing (although there are situations where this might not be welcomed by others), praying, and practicing mindfulness.

The information in this article is educational and is not intended as medical advice. It is a compilation of natural methods which have been effective for diminishing the symptoms of fibromyalgia and chronic fatigue syndrome in many individuals. It is not intended as diagnosis, treatment, of prescription for any disease or illness. The decision to use, or not to use, any of this information is the sole responsibility of the reader. Each person must make his or her own decisions regarding what is best for his or her health. If you believe you need medical advice and/or treatment, see your medical doctor or other duly licensed health care professional.

A Dozen Short-and-Sweet Things to Alleviate the Symptoms of Fibromyalgia and Chronic Fatigue

1. Enjoy the effects of mineral hot-springs at home.   The healing effects of the world's natural mineral springs are legendary, and for centuries, the wealthy have traveled great distances to partake. You can create a similar effect at home in your tub. Dissolve 1 cup of salt (any variety will do, Epsom salt or kitchen salt is fine) in a tub of comfortably hot water. While the water is running, get your radio or portable cassette player, put on some relaxation music, and light a candle or two to create relaxing atmosphere while you soak. If your tailbone or neck don't like the hardness of the tub, fold a towel to sit on, and another to place behind your neck to cushion these areas. Soak for about twenty minutes, or until the water begins to cool. Enjoy this treatment every six weeks or so; it will help draw toxins from the skin and superficial muscles, facilitate circulation, and help you relax and sleep better. Caution: extremely hot temperatures, such as hot-tubs, can actually "bake in" the toxins and contribute to achiness, so make your water a comfortable temperature Add a few drops of Lavender essential oil for relaxation, or Peppermint to feel more alert and awake.

2. Use skin-brushing to stimulate all the energetic meridians and lymphatic flows of the body. If your skin is extremely sensitive, start with a soft wash cloth, and do your skin brushing while you are lathered up in the shower. After two or three weeks, try a loofa sponge, with wet skin but without soap. Eventually work your way up to using a fairly stiff natural fiber brush, such as the kind used to scrub vegetables. You will be a pro when you can use the brush on dry skin! This simple procedure has numerous benefits for everyone, not just people who have fibromyalgia or chronic fatigue. It stimulates all the meridians, it moves the blood and lymphatic fluids, it helps oxygenate the blood (thus relieving fatigue and foggy-headed feelings and increasing energy level), and it helps the skin to discharge toxins and waste products. It also helps to keep the skin baby-soft by removing superficial layers of dead or dry skin cells.

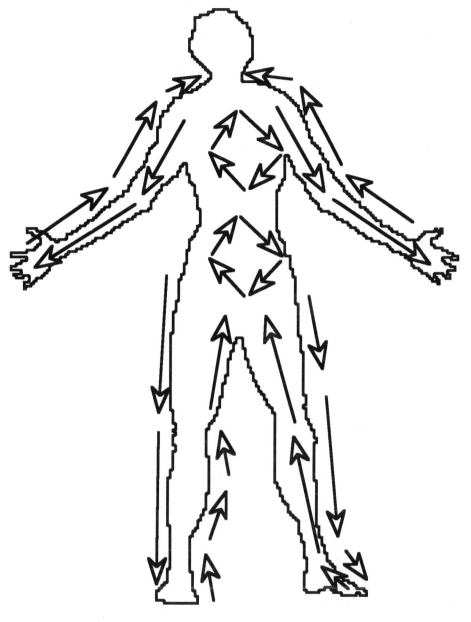

Skin Brushing Instructions

Hold your loofa or brush in the right hand and start with the chest area on the left side. All your brushing motions will be circular. Start by circular brushing the left chest area, then continue your circular motions down the inside surface (the palmar side) of the arm, all the way out to the hand and fingers. Then work your way up the outside of the arm, including the back of the wrist, elbow, and shoulder joints. Do the top of the shoulders and the back and sides of the neck. Switch the loofa to your left hand and repeat for the other arm. Next, do circular brushing all over the front of your torso, including the abdomen, rib area, and breasts.

Do your brushing in a clockwise motion, going down on the left side and upwards on the right side. Next, brush the hips, buttocks, and your low back area. Place the loofa in your left hand, and brush with circular strokes down the outer aspect of your left thigh and calf, then moving to the foot and ankle. If it is hard to bend over to reach that far, place your foot on the ledge of the bathtub. Be sure to get the sole of the foot also. Continue your circular brushing movements up the inside of the leg and thigh. Switch the loofa to the right hand to treat the right leg. The whole procedure should be brisk and quick, covering the whole body in 2-3 minutes. If you do this regularly every other day (or more often if you wish) you will notice an improvement in your energy level and stamina after a few weeks. Its also a great pick-me-up if you are feeling tired, but have something you must do.

3. **The Broomstick stretch:** Find a broom stick, mop handle, yard-stick, or similar long, narrow, solid object. While standing, grasp the broom stick in front of you with your hands as far apart as possible and palms facing the wall behind you, elbows relaxed. The task is to get the broomstick behind you any way you can, without letting go of your grip; then get it back to the front. If your upper body is very tight and achey, start with three sets (1 set = front to back, then back to front). Work your way up to 10 sets. As a special treat, when you finish, use the broomstick like a rolling pin to massage the tops of your shoulders, neck, upper back, and shoulder blades. Feels great, and it will really help with upper body tension.

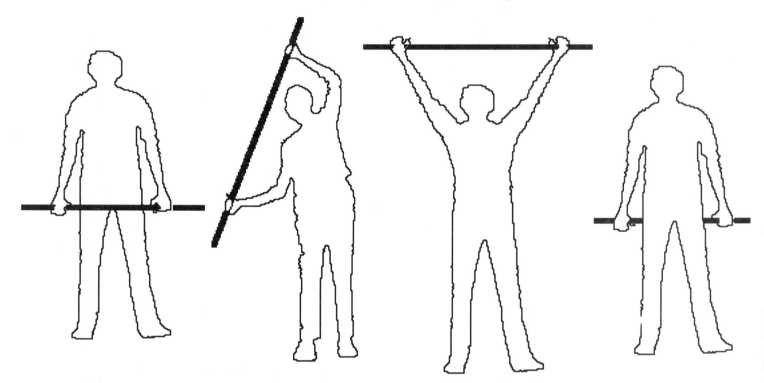

4. **Tennis Ball Acupressure.** Ask a tennis player for four well-used tennis balls. (Brand new ones are likely to be much too firm). Then get a pair of old socks, and put two tennis balls in each sock. Secure the open end with a rubber band or tie a knot in the sock. There should be about a half inch of empty space between the tennis balls so they can move a bit inside the sock. Now lie down on a bed or sofa (a surface which has some "give" to it) and place the tennis balls behind your neck, between your shoulder blades, under your low back area, or wherever it hurts. Adjust your body position until you get the balls in just the right spot. Then relax your weight onto the balls to give self-acupressure. In most cases, 5 minutes on one spot will be plenty to give a noticable release in the area. Great for those sore achey spots that are difficult to reach!

5. Relax with herbal tea before bedtime. Chamomille is a time honored natural relaxant which makes a delicious tea to use before bedtime. There are several popular brands of herbal tea featuring chamomille as the chief ingredient. Fix a cup about an hour before you plan to retire for the evening, then just sip and wind down slowly for bedtime.

6. Breathe. One of the most simple natural methods for increasing your energy and relieving fatigue is to breathe deeply. When there is frequent or continuous fatigue, it is a sign that the blood is overly acidic. The fastest, easiest, and most healthful way to shift the blood to a more alkaline condition is to do relaxed deep breathing. Sit down on the edge of a firm chair, such as a kitchen chair, with both feet flat on the floor. Straighten your spine so your head is balanced above your shoulders, giving a free and clear airway. Place your hands on your thighs. (If sitting is very uncomfortable, lie down on a firm mattress or on the floor. Your legs should be straight and uncrossed, and your hands at your sides or resting comfortably over your navel. Close your eyes, and focus your attention on your breathing, first noticing how you breathe when you aren't doing anything special about it. Then shift to a deep breathing pattern, which is slow and feels as though the breath goes all the way into your abdomen. Let your tummy expand and contract with each breath. Allow your shoulders to relax and drop. Pause for a second or two between breaths. Start with 12 deep breaths at each session. When that becomes easier and feels natural, then go to 24, then 36. This is good to do upon rising every morning, and sometime during the afternoon to give you some renewed energy for the rest of the day.

7. Go outside for at least 10-15 minutes every day. Take off your sunglasses to let the natural full-spectrum light enter your eyes, where it can stimulate the pineal gland. Research into the effects of light on healing shows that depression is often alleviated significantly by simply exposing oneself to natural daylight. In addition, sunlight stimulates the production of vitamin D in the skin, which is much healthier than relying on synthetic additives. While you are out there, enjoy something of nature. Even if you live in an urban environment, you can probably find a flower or other plant to enjoy, watch cloud formations in the sky, or watch children playing. Spending some time out-of-doors is especially important for sedentary people. Just the openness, the bigger space of the outdoors helps to create a feeling of more space and openness within.

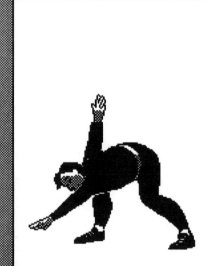

8. Stretch. Many fibromyalgia patients report that daily stretching does more to relieve aches and stiffness than any other thing that they do for themselves. There are numerous video cassettes available which can be purchased in video stores for around $20. Select one on Yoga or stretching which is directed at relaxation and/or pain relief. Many people tend to do these exercises more regularly when they can do them at home, in privacy, without having to fit a class and driving time into their schedule. Others do better if they have a structured class time and fellow exercisers to give moral support and social contact, so they prefer to go to a health club, fitness center, or Yoga studio for their exercise time.

9. Begin to "regularize" your day. Onset of FMS or CFIDS is often preceded by a time of chaos, confusion and unpredictability or crisis in life. Sometimes this is a single situation or series of situations such as death in the family, job change, family or relationship problems or accident. Some people live their entire life as a series of crises and chaotic events. Even in robust health, the body prefers regularity in its activities, and for fibromyalgia and chronic fatigue, this can make all the difference. It helps to put YOU back in the driver's seat of your life, instead of having outside influences pushing and pulling you about. Areas to look at, and begin to make changes, are regular meal times (sit down at the table, eat in a relaxed way, appreciating your food and welcome the nourishment you are receiving), time of arising in the morning, time of retiring at night, bath time, exercise time, and relaxation periods during the day. If you have been letting your day be controlled by hectic activities of family members, phone interruptions, etc, take back your control, even if you seem to be "old maidish" or if it inconveniences your kids or spouse. They will adjust in a short time, especially if you keep your sense of humor and keep it light.

10. Do something nice for someone else every day. With chronic problems such as fibromyalgia or fatigue, it is very easy to become obsessed with one's own difficulties, pain, and so on. When we move our attention outside of ourselves, and do a sincerely motivated caring act for someone else, it brings pleasure and joy which can often counteract much of our own discomfort. Every healer I have ever known, from mental health counselors, to massage therapists, to chiropractic physicians, knows that the most powerful way to self-healing is to assist others with their healing. In helping another to heal, we heal ourselves.

11. Eat whole foods. You don't need to become a vegetarian in order to clean up your diet. Just eat foods that really are food. Real foods are things that were alive recently, or are still alive (whole grains can sprout and grow, potatoes and onions and garlic can put out shoots even in the vegetable bin of your fridge.) Snack foods, artificial things like soda pop, and packaged or convenience foods are a long way from the concept of whole and natural. Purchase foods fresh and make friends with a gardner and a fisherman who would share a bumper crop with your family!   In addition to the health benefits of eating whole and natural foods, you may find that your grocery bill goes down as you eliminate the refined, processed, and chemicalized products; they are some of the most high-priced items in the store!   Center your plate around nourishing vegetables, grains, beans, and fruits. Select poultry or fish much more than red meats, and minimize or eliminate dairy products if you wish to increase your energy level and reduce your muscle aches and depression. Eliminate aspartame (nutrasweet, equal, diet drinks).

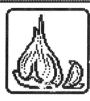

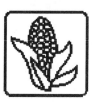

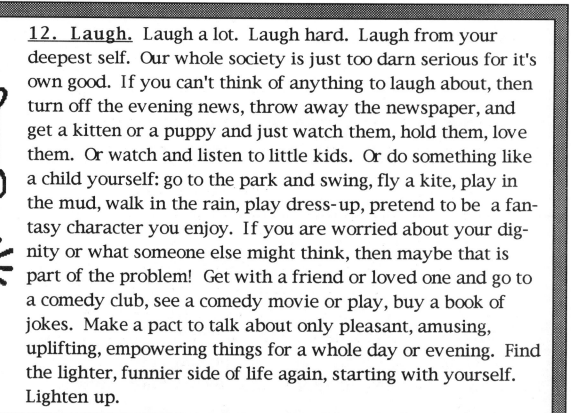

12. Laugh. Laugh a lot. Laugh hard. Laugh from your deepest self. Our whole society is just too darn serious for it's own good. If you can't think of anything to laugh about, then turn off the evening news, throw away the newspaper, and get a kitten or a puppy and just watch them, hold them, love them. Or watch and listen to little kids. Or do something like a child yourself: go to the park and swing, fly a kite, play in the mud, walk in the rain, play dress-up, pretend to be a fantasy character you enjoy. If you are worried about your dignity or what someone else might think, then maybe that is part of the problem! Get with a friend or loved one and go to a comedy club, see a comedy movie or play, buy a book of jokes. Make a pact to talk about only pleasant, amusing, uplifting, empowering things for a whole day or evening. Find the lighter, funnier side of life again, starting with yourself. Lighten up.

FREQUENTLY ASKED QUESTIONS

Q: IS IT REALLY POSSIBLE TO TOTALLY RECOVER FROM FIBROMYALGIA AND CHRONIC FATIGUE?

A: It is possible to make great improvement, and some people recover so that fatigue or pain are insignificant factors in their everyday lives. This is what I mean by recovery. Such people have to maintain constant vigilance in their lifestyle choices, food, exercise, and mental/emotional attitudes. Most continue to work with a holistic practitioner (massage or shiatsu therapist, acupuncturist, naturopath, chiropractor, or holistic medical doctor) on a regular basis. Fibromyalgia and chronic fatigue are chronic problems, and can flare under extremes of stress, exhaustion, or when a person reverts to former unhealthy habits. Put your attention on improving to the highest degree you can.

Q: I'VE HAD SO MUCH DIFFICULTY FINDING A PHYSICIAN WHO WILL WORK WITH ME. SEVERAL THAT I HAVE SEEN DON'T SEEM TO THINK I HAVE A REAL PHYSICAL DISORDER. WHY DON'T THEY BELIEVE ME?

A. Physicians are trained to diagnose illness primarily based on lab tests, MRI's, and other technological methods.   These tests can help identify problems such as thyroid imbalance or blood sugar disorders which can produce some of the same symptoms as fibromyalgia and chronic fatigue. So far, there is no lab test or scan that helps the doctor diagnose fibromyalgia and chronic fatigue. Also, the symptoms vary widely among different individuals, some having very mild symptoms and others almost totally disabled. fibromyalgia and chronic fatigue are "functional disorders". This means the body systems aren't working very well and the whole person is affected. Stress and unhealthy lifestyle cause body physiology to work in abnormal ways, often leading to symptoms.   Medical science is just beginning to recognize and train doctors in a whole new field called "functional medicine". This may be the medical approach which will ultimately prove most beneficial for those with fibromyalgia and chronic fatigue and other functional disorders. If you can find a doctor who has received training in this field, they will work with diet, supplements, and other methods similar to practitioners who are trained in holistic health care.

Q. ALL THE DOCTOR WANTS TO DO IS GIVE ME PILLS TO CONTROL MY SYMPTOMS.   SOME OF THE MEDICATIONS HELPED FOR AWHILE, BUT THEN THEY EITHER CREATE A NEW SIDE EFFECT, OR STOP WORKING. I'VE EVEN HAD SOME MEDICATIONS THAT I COULDN'T TAKE BECAUSE THEY MADE ME FEEL LIKE A ZOMBIE, OR MADE SOME SYMPTOMS WORSE. ANYWAY, I DON'T WANT TO TAKE DRUGS THE REST OF MY LIFE!   THEY ARE EXPENSIVE, AND SOME HAVE UNDESIRABLE SIDE EFFECTS! WHAT SHOULD I DO?

A: There is a place for chemical medications   in the management of fibromyalgia and chronic fatigue for some people, and they can help by jump-starting a person's physiology so the person can begin to look at lifestyle changes and other things they can do. For example, anti-depressants for a few months can help a person move from "non-functioning" to a state where they can begin to actively do things to change their condition.

Medical schools train doctors to adjust physiological problems with medicine. Very few conventional physicians are trained in nutrition, stress management, therapeutic exercise, meditation, or other natural methods. Those who are have sought out such training due to a sense of needing more to offer their patients. If you cannot find a holistically oriented medical doctor, you might find that a naturopathic or chiropractic physician or oriental medical doctor has more to offer of what you are asking for. You can use conventional and alternative care together as needed.

Q. WILL MY HEALTH INSURANCE PAY FOR THERAPIES SUCH AS MASSAGE, SHIATSU, ACUPUNCTURE OR HERBS?

A. You will have to check with your health insurance provider or the benefits office where you work. In most cases the answer will be "no". Health insurance is designed to pay for "medical or surgical" treatment, and alternative and complementary therapies generally do not meet those criteria. Some coverage will pay for sessions of physical therapy or chiropractic care, but many are even limiting these options.

I recommend you strive to find the money in your budget to allocate for your visits to a practitioner. Your health needs to become a major priority if you want to get better, and paying for services out-of-pocket may be necessary as part of that commitment. It may require some sacrifices in the short term but yields long term benefits. Many people find that if they can reduce some of their medications, medical co-payments and other expenses, they have enough to pay for the visits to their holistic practitioner. For many people, "paying their own way" increases motivation and commitment to a program. What you pay for yourself will hold greater value to you.

Q: MY LIFE HAS BEEN TURNED UPSIDE DOWN BY THIS ILLNESS. I'VE HAD TO QUIT MY JOB, AND MOST OF MY FRIENDS DON'T CALL ANY MORE BECAUSE I'VE TURNED THEM DOWN SO MANY TIMES. MY FAMILY DOESN'T UNDERSTAND. HOW CAN I GET MY OLD LIFE BACK?

A: Chronic illness is a transformational journey. We never like it when we are in the transformational stages because we have to uproot ourselves from old familiar ways of doing things and enter a new way of life. I'm sorry to say it, but your old way of life is probably gone forever. There are two paths before you now, and you have free will to choose which way to go. You can allow your illness to take over and control your life, or you can take control of your life even though you have a chronic illness. If you are willing to do whatever it takes to get better and adapt to changes, then the second path is the one you will ultimately choose. It will bring new friends, new ways to make a living, new self-image, and much more. You may even become a positive role model for your family members, who one day, may be faced with a health challenge as you are now.

Q: WHAT DID I DO TO DESERVE THIS? I'VE HEARD THAT "WE CREATE OUR OWN REALITY" BUT I DON'T THINK ANYONE WOULD BRING THIS KIND OF MISERY AND PAIN INTO THEIR LIFE ON PURPOSE. AM I BEING PUNISHED FOR BEING A BAD PERSON?

A: No, you are not being punished. Health challenges eventually confront everyone. The physical body can take a lot, and is meant to be a sturdy vehicle for our mind and spirit, but people come into the world with different physical vulnerabilities. For some, health challenges may not appear until old age; others have them while young or middle-aged.

"We Create Our Own Reality" is a spiritual truth that is part of every major spiritual tradition. It is meant to teach us responsibility for all our choices and actions. Every action has multiple outcomes, both short term and long term. For example, a person may decide to work two or three jobs to meet a financial crisis, but down the road there will be a price to pay physically, emotionally, or mentally. Each time we make a choice, we activate certain potential outcomes, and deactivate others. Part of life's process is learning what outcomes may develop from our choices. Some of these choices may even occur at a level beyond our physical life and personality awareness. When a person develops a physical illness, it may be an outcome of earlier choices, or it may be a starting point where she/he can begin to create the outcomes that will shape her/his future by the attitudes she/he holds and the decisions she/he makes.

Q: I WENT TO A SUPPORT GROUP THINKING I WOULD FIND ANSWERS, BUT INSTEAD IT REALLY GOT ME UPSET. SOME PEOPLE SAID I COULD END UP IN A WHEELCHAIR. OTHERS SAID I WILL ONLY GET WORSE AND THERE IS NOTHING THAT CAN BE DONE FOR ME. I FEEL LIKE I'VE BEEN GIVEN A LIFE SENTENCE. WHAT SHOULD I BELIEVE?

A. Different support groups have different personalities. It depends on the leaders and the people who attend regularly. Some groups could more aptly be called "similar problem clubs" or "gloom-and-doom societies". These will only support attendees in staying stuck and miserable, increasing their fear and suffering. Some people with fibromyalgia and chronic fatigue have started their own recovery-oriented support groups. Three to ten people who are committed to getting better can be a very effective group. A small group can meet at members' homes and be a forum for exploration of health issues, including stress, emotional, and family issues. One good way to start is by group study of relevant books. Many titles are given in the section on "Lifestyle and Nutrition Based Recovery" earlier in this chapter. Use books to generate discussion topics and explore things you can do for yourself. Members can take turns being the meeting facilitator to keep the conversation on track. Have an organizational meeting to find out everyone's interests and concerns, and select a format and schedule for future meetings.

Q: HOW DO I CHOOSE A HOLISTIC PRACTITIONER? I DON'T HAVE THE TIME, ENERGY OR MONEY TO TRY A LOT OF DIFFERENT THINGS.

A: Recommendations from friends, associates, or other practitioners is the best way. Support groups may be able to help with this. If you don't know anyone who can recommend a therapist, you may have to call several and ask about their experience with fibromyalgia and chronic fatigue. Ask them what sort of therapies they use. Ask them if they would be willing to have one of their existing clients call you and share their experiences.

Q: HOW DO I START? I'M BEGINNING TO REALIZE THERE ARE SO MANY THINGS I COULD BE DOING, ITS OVERWHELMING!! I REALLY LIKE THE IDEA OF LIFESTYLE CHANGES, BUT I DON'T HAVE MUCH ENERGY TO ORGANIZE AND FIGURE THIS OUT.

A: Start by picking things that would be easy for you to do in your present condition. For example, daily exposure to natural sunlight, or starting new supplements are easy for many people. Work with that for two to four weeks, and then add another change. Exercise can be very simple if you choose walking or a few minutes of mini-trampoline each day. Start slowly and increase gradually. Pick something that feels attractive to you, and that you would be willing to make a commitment to. Keep it simple.

Q: I WAS DOING REALLY WELL FOR A FEW WEEKS. I THOUGHT I WAS FINALLY ON THE ROAD TO RECOVERY. THEN WE HAD A BIG SCARE ABOUT LAYOFFS AT MY JOB, AND NOW I'M RIGHT BACK WHERE I STARTED! HAVE I FAILED TO DO SOMETHING RIGHT?

A. Fibromyalgia and chronic fatigue symptoms seem to get worse under stress, and improve when things are going smoothly, independently of all the other good things you are doing for yourself. The stress at your job probably triggered a flare-up of your symptoms. Stress, exhaustion, even weather changes can affect these two syndromes. A flare can last a few days, or even a few weeks for some individuals. Resume your good habits and lifestyle changes and work with stress management tools to deal with stress that comes into your life. Many people learn to identify the start of a flare and take measures to keep it minimal, for example getting extra sleep, taking time off, having an extra session with their body therapist, talking to friends for support. Most people find that each time they cycle through flares, getting back to a good state becomes easier. Look for your overall trend of improvement, not the little day-to-day fluctuations. Like the stock market, there are ups and downs, but the overall trend is upward.

Appendix 1

Clinic Intake Form
Fibromyalgia and Chronic Fatigue Syndrome

Client Name _____ Date _____

Chief complaint

Secondary complaints

When was the onset?

Sudden or gradual onset?

Circumstances of onset

Head symptoms: sinus, ears ringing, throat, TMJ, tongue pain, lymph nodes, eyes, headache, neck pain, vision problems?

Chest symptoms: Palpitations, cough, mucus, catches colds easily, cardiac problems, asthma, respiratory allergies, shallow breathing, tender in upper ribs/lymphatic areas, breast fibroids?

Digestion: Nausea, distension, ulcers, gas or bloating, diarrhea, constipation, sluggish digestion, hiatal hernia, irritable bowel, frequency of elimination?

Urinary: Frequency of urination, pale or dark urine, infections, burning, incontinence, bladder dropping, kidney stones, unexplained low back pain?

Female: age of first menses, ease of menstruation, regularity of menstruation, PMS, pregnancies, (how many, how long ago, and ease of pregnancy and delivery), menopause?

Male: prostate, GI tract problems? Discomfort on urination, incomplete urination, frequent or night-time urination?

<u>Skin and Nails:</u> Dry, moist, itchy, rashes, bruises, brittle nails, varicose veins?

<u>Musculo-skeletal:</u> quality of pain, location of pain, duration of pain, continuous or intermittent, morning stiffness, factors which aggravate or diminish pain; muscles, joints, spine?

<u>Sleep:</u> how many hours per night, quality, difficulty falling asleep, waking in the night, time of waking, feeling restored in the morning, difficult rising?

<u>Temperature:</u> tendency to chills or cold limbs, tendency to feel hot all over or in extremities, hot flashes, night sweats

<u>Psychological:</u> dominant emotions, depression, anxiety, dreams, memory, concentration, ease of planning, decision making, self-motivation

<u>Medical History:</u> accidents, injuries, surgeries, illness, medications (Rx and OTC), vaccinations; any correlated with time of onset of FMS or CFIDS

<u>Previous Therapy:</u> What has helped; what has not helped;

<u>Stress and Character:</u> What are the major stressor in this person's life? How are their stress-coping mechanisms? Are they stress-hardy? Are they self-efficacious? Do they have empowering beliefs?

<u>Pulse, Tongue, and Other Observations:</u>

<u>Homework and Client Education:</u> What areas are they willing to explore?   Do they have interest in exercise, Yoga, Tai Chi, nutrition, meditation, herbs, aromatherapy, supplements, homeopathy, etc. Would they like for you to recommend a book or a class on any of these subjects?

<u>Other comments or correlations:</u>

Appendix 2

Seven Signs of Health in Chinese Medicine

1)   I have excellent physical and mental <u>stamina and resilience</u>; I easily <u>follow through</u> to complete tasks and projects; I do not normally experience fatigue. (Maximum 5 points).

2) I have a <u>good appetite</u> for food, life, personal growth, change, study, and learning (maximum 5 points).

3) I experience <u>good sleep</u>; I can fall asleep quickly and wake up refreshed, relaxed, and centered; my dreams relate to future events and problem-solving. (maximum 5 points)

4) I have <u>good memory</u>. I can remember names and numbers as well as faces, images and melodies. (maximum 10 points).

5) I am <u>always cheerful and pleasant</u>; I never get angry; grousing or complaining are not like me. (Maximum 10 points).

6) <u>Decision-making</u> is smooth and easy for me; I have <u>quick reflexes</u> and do not have accidents. (Maximum 10 points).

7) I experience and express <u>appreciation and gratitude</u>; I have a sense of <u>higher purpose</u> and being part of something bigger than myself; I <u>acknowledge problems as opportunities</u>; I never have to lie to myself or others (Maximum 55 points).

Appendix 3

Living In Harmony With the Natural Laws

1. Eat only foods that are alive or have been alive recently.

2. Get adequate rest, a regular amount of sleep every night

3. Move every joint and muscle in your body every day.

4. Find a balance between work and play.

5. Find a balance between activity and relaxation.

6. Meditate and/or pray every day.

7. Have a creative outlet for your personal expression.

8. Interact with animals and plants on a regular basis.

9. Expose yourself to natural sunlight every day.

10. Drink plenty of pure water every day.

11. Share your life with supportive and loving people.

12. Culture mindfulness in all your daily activities. Live in the moment.   Today is all you have.

13. Be of service.

14. See the humorous side of life.

15. Mourn your losses, lick your wounds, and then move on with life. Everything that happens is potentially rich with learning and personal or spiritual development.

16. Work toward appropriate bonding and boundaries with the people in your life. Only engage in sithations that are win-win.

17. Develop self-mastery.

Appendix 4
Health Goals Planning Worksheet

Part 1. Please write three to five personal health goals. Think them through carefully. Make them as clear and specific as possible and include a time frame in which you plan to accomplish each goal. Identify the benefits for you, and determine whether the goal is appropriate for you. Write a few words about what this will do for you. Include at least one goal for physical, one for mental/emotional, and one for spiritual well-being (refer to lists below). Your goals should be appropriate for your age and condition, and they should be appealing to you. Examples:

"I will lose twenty pounds in four months, and I will look better and have more energy" or "I will build up to three miles of brisk walking four times per week, by April 1, and this will increase my stamina for hiking/ biking" or "I will work with my doctor to eliminate 'X' medication by the end of the year, and this will reduce expenses, get rid of side effects, and help me learn natural ways of eliminating symptom 'Z', or "I will take a workshop once each quarter on health or stress management", or "I will change my work load so I am working a maximum of forty hours per week with two days off. This will reduce stress, allow me to get more sleep, and spend more time with the family. I will do this in a three month period."

1._____

2._____

3._____

4._____

5._____

Part 2. Now that you know where you are, and where you want to go, next you need to determine what you are going to do all along the way. First you need methods and materials. Perhaps you need to buy a pair of walking shoes or hand weights or a mini-trampoline, or you need a plan for weight reduction. Maybe you need to find a class or reading materials. Some goals will require money, some will not. Find ways to structure the goals so your resources of time and money can support them.

Then begin to work with your space and time frames to determine where you need to be by certain times. For example, to lose twenty pounds in four months, you will average five pounds per month. If you want to meditate, you need to set aside the time and prepare a place where you can be undisturbed for your meditation period. For each goal, map out your plans. Below is a sample of items to include. Use extra paper as needed for planning.

HEALTH GOALS PLANNING WORKSHEET

Use separate a sheet for each one of your health goals. Adapt the suggestions given here to best meet your own situation.

Date: _____

Goal:

_____

What this will do for me:

_____

_____

Impact on others (family, co-workers, friends):

_____

_____

Materials I need:

_____

What I need to purchase and estimated cost:

_____

Resources I already have or are free (library, internet etc.):

_____

_____

Resource people and courses:

_____

_____

Reading or study resource materials (books, videos, magazines, web sites):

_____

_____

Space requirements

_____

Methods I will use

_____

_____

Time each day/week devoted to goal (include reading and learning activities)

_____

Starting measurement

_____

Benchmarks along the way (target and actual):

	Target	Actual		Target	Actual
Week 1	_____	_____	Week 5	_____	_____
Week 2	_____	_____	Week 6	_____	_____
Week 3	_____	_____	Week 7	_____	_____
Week 4	_____	_____	Week 8	_____	_____

Examples of Healthful Practices for Body, Mind, and Spirit

<u>Physical</u>	<u>Mental/Emotional</u>	<u>Spiritual</u>
Stretching/Yoga	Counselling	Prayer
Swimming/ Jogging	Support Groups	Meditation
Walking/ Hiking	Twelve-step programs	Past-life work
Tai Chi/ Qi Gong	Neuro-Linguistic	Zen/ Dharma practices
Acupuncture	Programming(NLP)	Course in Miracles
Water/ Step Aerobics	Hypnotherapy	Spirituality groups
Breath work	Psychotherapy	Women's studies
Shiatsu/ Massage	Dream work	Men's studies
Dance	Gestalt therapy	Drumming circles
Nutritional	Astrology	I Ching
Supplements	Addiction recovery	Tarot
Whole Foods	Body-mind therapy	Metaphysics
Medicinal Herbs	Journal writing	Spiritual Healing
Weight Training	Cognitive therapy	Native American Ritual
Fitness Workouts	Gay/Lesbian support	Nature/ Wilderness
Treadmill/ Ski Machine	Self-help books	Chanting
Sports and Games	Co-dependency books	Mantra
Mountain Biking	Internet research	Intuitive Development

Appendix 5
Meridians of Traditional Chinese Medicine

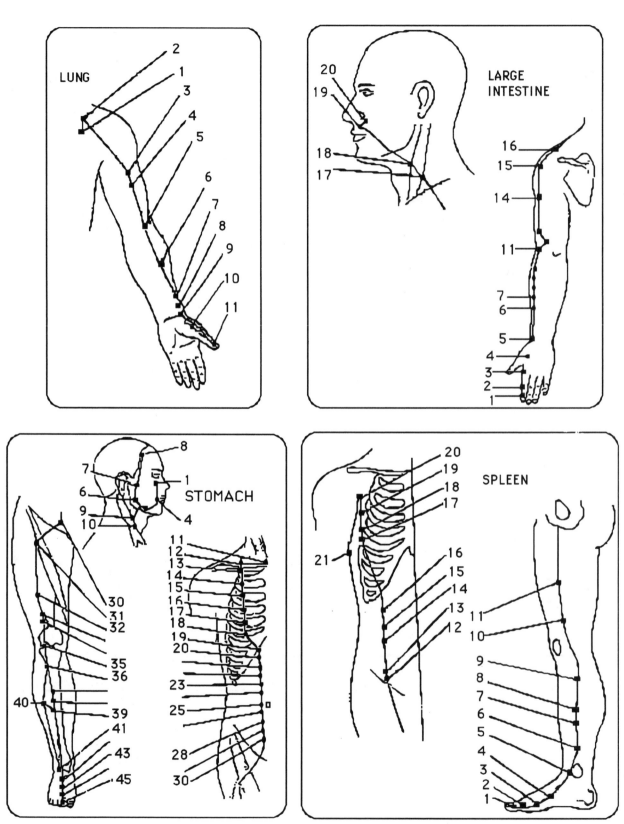

175

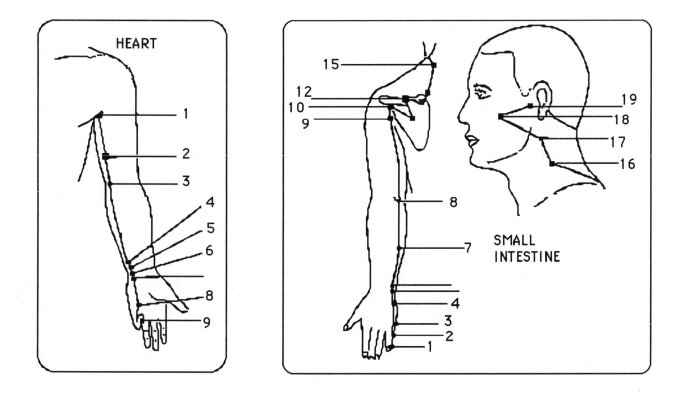

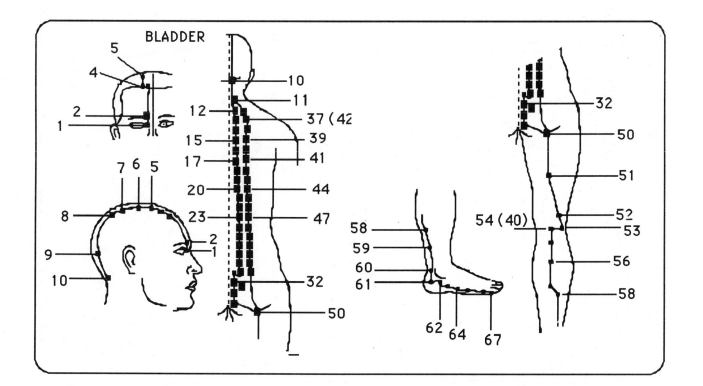

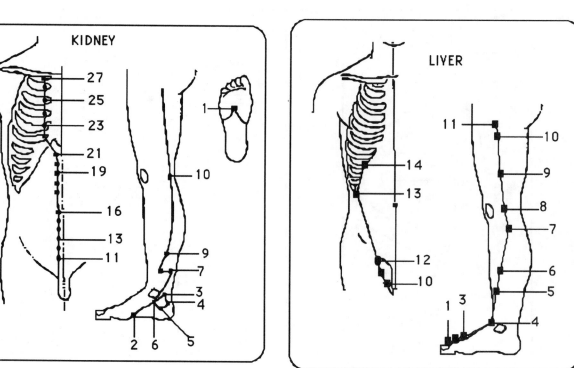

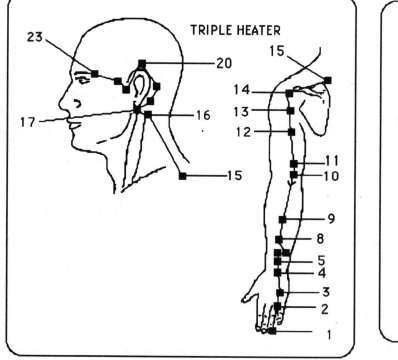

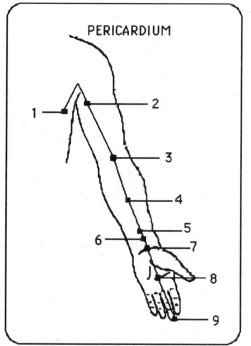

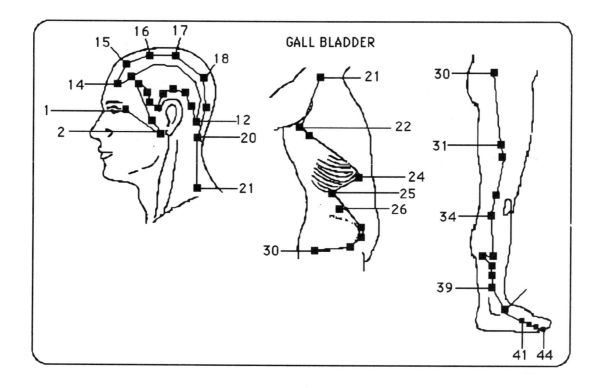

GALL BLADDER

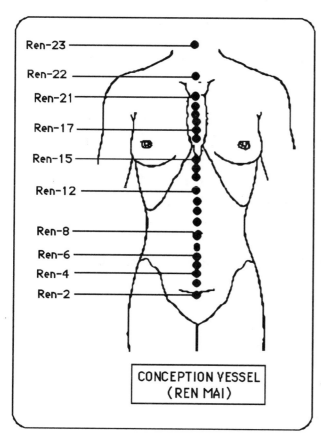

CONCEPTION VESSEL
(REN MAI)

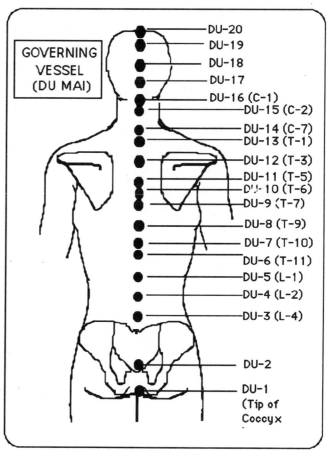

GOVERNING VESSEL (DU MAI)

Appendix 6

Cleansing Diet for Colon and Lymphatic System

Day 1: Eat fruit, all you want such as apples, berries, watermelon, pears, cherries, but no bananas. Drink plenty of pure spring water

Day 2: Drink all the herbal teas you want, such as chamomile, raspberry, spearmint, hyssop. If you desire to sweeten the teas, use only pure maple syrup. Drink plenty of pure spring water.

Day 3: Eat all the vegetables you want, such as carrots, celery, cabbage, green beans, onions, broccoli, cauliflower. Have them raw or steamed.
Drink plenty of pure spring water

Day 4: Prepare a pot of vegetable broth using cauliflower, cabbage, onion, green pepper, broccoli, parsley, or whatever you have on hand. Season only with sea salt or Herbal seasoning. Use filtered or spring water to prepare the broth. Drink only this rich mineral broth all day.

On the first day the colon is cleansed. The second day the body releases toxins, salt, and excessive calcium deposits from the muscles, tissues and organs. The third day the digestive tract is supplied with healthful, mineral-rich fiber. The fourth day the blood, lymph and organs are mineralized.

It is also recommended to do the following in conjunction with this four-day program:

- Contrast shower (cold-hot-cold) each day
- Skin brushing after the shower
- Castor oil packs on colon and/or liver at bed time each night of the cleanse

Appendix 7
About The Author:
Sunny Cooper, M.S., O.B.T.

Sunny Cooper has been studying traditional Chinese medicine and oriental bodywork since 1987. She holds degrees from Purdue University and University of Michigan, with background in the natural sciences. She graduated from Blue Cliff School of Therapeutic Massage in Kenner, Louisiana in 1989. She is a Certified Instructor for the American Oriental Bodywork Therapy Association (AOBTA) and is Board Certified in Oriental Bodywork by the National Certification Commission for Acupuncture and Oriental Medicine (NCCAOM).

From 1990 to 1993 she was official sports-massage therapist for the Gayle Hatch Olympic Weight-lifting Team in Baton Rouge, Louisiana. She was a presenter at the 1996 AOBTA national convention in Chicago, and travels across the country to do workshops and seminars in Chinese medicine and bodywork. She has a clinical practice in Ogden and Bountiful, Utah. She is a Master Practitioner of Neuro-Linguistic Programming and is certified in Ericksonian hypnotherapy. She conducts oriental bodywork trainings from beginner to advanced for massage therapists, bodyworkers, and other health care practitioners. She is an adjunct faculty member at Weber State University, teaching courses in School of Nursing.

Sunny Cooper is approved by the National Certification Board for Therapeutic Massage and Bodywork (NCBTMB) as a continuing education provider. She teaches classes and workshops on fibromyalgia and chronic fatigue as well as other topics in Chinese medical theory and practice and holistic health care. Interested schools, organizations or practitioners may arrange for a workshop in your area. Contact the author in care of the publisher of this book: Life Circles Publications, 965 East 28th Street, Ogden UT 84403, phone (801)-782-2993, Email ShuPoint@aol.com.

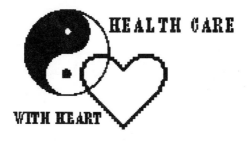

Glossary

Acupressure- "acupunture without needles". Stimulation of the points and meridians by touch, usually with medium to firm pressure.

Acupuncture- insertion of fine needles into the points to produce shifts in the flow or distribution of the body's energy.

Acute illness or injury- an illness or injury of short duration which resolves completely. Examples are the common cold or a sprained ankle.

Acutherapy- therapy given by stimulating the acupoints and/or meridians of the body. Acupuncture, acupressure, shiatsu, and tuina are examples.

Aromatherapy- therapy done using essential oils of plants which have healing properties. (See chapter 10)

Ayurvedic medicine- the ancient traditional medicine of India. Includes the use of herbs, food, exercise, meditation, massage, and lifestyle change to improve health.

Bilateral- occurring on both sides of the body. For example, all the main meridians of the body are bilateral, being present on both right and left sides.

Blood- in Chinese medicine Blood includes many body fluids including blood, lymph, and cellular fluid.

Chronic Illness- illness or injury lasting a long time. Usually a condition which has been present for six months or longer is considered to be chronic.

Coccyx- the tailbone.

Craniosacral Therapy- a system of therapy involving subtle hands-on manipulation of the head and sacrum and other body areas to improve the flow of cerebrospinal fluid, release fascial restrictions in the body, and release restrictions in the sutures of the cranial bones.

Cupping- a technique from Chinese medicine in which glass or plastic cups are evacuated and placed on an area of congestion in order to relieve pain and stiffness in the area.

Cure- complete disappearance of a disease.

Dan Tien- a major energy center in the body located in the pelvic cavity just below the umbilicus.

Dark Night of the Soul- a phrase coined by St. John of the Cross referring to a period of feeling isolated and detached from other people and everyday life during spiritual work.

Deficiency- a lack of something. In Chinese medicine, Blood or Qi may be deficient, resulting in symptoms.

Eight Extra Vessels- eight special meridians used in acupuncture and acupressure to adjust the deeper balance of energy within the body.

Essential Oils- substances with medicinal properties which are distilled from plants and used in aromatherapy.

Extraordinary Vessels- see "eight extra vessels"

Five Elements- a model for working with patterns of observed phenomena in Chinese medicine. The five elements are Fire, Earth, Metal, Wood, and Water. In this system all five are interdependent.

Governing Vessel- a major meridian on the back surface of the body, related to the brain and central nervous system.

Healing- transformation in a positive manner. Moving toward better harmony of body, mind, and spirit.

Iatrogenic- symptoms or illness caused by medical or therapeutic intervention. For example, side effects of drug, or disability caused by surgery.

Jin Shin Do- a style of acupressure integrating Jungian psychotherapy with stimulation of points on the eight extraordinary vessels.

Lymphatic system- a body system which serves as part of the immune system and moves fluids, immune cells, and waste products through the body.

Lymphotome- a surface region of the body in which the lymph drains in a particular direction.

Meridians- pathways on and in the body in which the vital energy or Qi flows.

Moxibustion- a technique in Chinese medicine in which heat is applied for therapeutic effects.

Neurolymphatic Reflex points- points on the body surface which can be massaged to stimulate the flow of lymph.

Palpation- examination by touch or pressing.

Paradigm- a system of thinking

Parasympathetic Nervous System- the portion of the nervous system which produces the relaxation response.

Pernicious Influence- factors which cause disharmony in the body. In Chinese medicine these are Heat, Cold, Wind, Damp, and Dry.

Physiotherapy- therapeutic modalities which can include touch, passive or active exercise, electrical stimulation, massage, and other methods to produce beneficial changes in the body.

Prone- face-down postition.

Qi- (also Chi and Ki)- the vital energy of Chinese medicine.

Qi Gong- a Chinese system of exercise used to promote health which involves use of movement, balance, breathing, mental focus, and meditation.

Reflex area- an area on the body which is connected to another area and can be used as an indicator of conditions in the related area. For example, foot reflexology uses areas on the feet to assess and balance all the organs and regions of the body.

Sacrum- The large triangular bone at the back of the hips, below the lumbar spine and above the coccyx (tailbone).

Shen- In Chinese medicine, the "spirit" or "mind".

Shiatsu- Japanese acupressure massage

Stagnation- A condition in which something is not moving freely as it should.

Structural Imbalance- an irregularity in the body's structure which may cause symptoms. Example: scoliosis, or curvature of the spine, may cause muscle pain, headaches, or impairment of organ function.

Supine- face-up position.

Sympathetic Nervous System- the portion of the nervous system responsible for the "fight or flight" response.

Tai Chi- a Chinese system of therapeutic exercise involving graceful controlled movement, mental focus and breathing in a pre-arranged dance-like form.

Taoism- a philosophical system from ancient China which recommends living a lifestyle of moderation and harmony with nauture.

Tender points- a group of eighteen points used by physicians in the diagnosis of fibromyalgia. The points were standardized by the American College of Rheumatologists in 1990.

Trigger points- neuromuscular regions in the muscles which, when activated, can cause local and referred pain. Releasing trigger points by massage techniques can reduce or alleviate pain and discomfort generated by the active trigger point.

Tuina- a system of Chinese massage used in hospitals and clinics in China.

Vital Substances- in Chinese medicine, the fluids of the body including Qi, Blood, Essence, and Shen.

Yin and Yang- in Chinese medicine, the two fundamental forces in nature; direction of energy movement.

Zang Fu- in Chinese medicine, the Organs of the body.

References

Affleck J. ME(CFIDS): a Vaccination Link? http://chetday.com/janecfids/html

Allen AD. Is RA27/3 Rubella immunization a cause of chronic fatigue? Med Hypotheses 1988 Nov; 27(3):217-20.

Ahles TA, Khan SA,Yunus MB, Spiegel DA, Masi AT. Psychiatric Status of patients with primary fibromyalgia, patients with rheumatoid arthritis, and subjects without pain: a blind comparison of DSM-III diagnoses. Am. J. Psychiatry 1991; 148(12): 1721-6.

American College of Rheumatology. WWW.Rheumatology.org.

Aspartame websites: http://www.dorway.com; http://www.health-today.net/aspartame.htm

Bandura, A. 1977. Self-Efficacy: toward a unifying theory of behavioral change. Psychological Review Mar 84(2):191-215.

Beinfield, Harriet, L.Ac. and Korngold, Efrem, L.Ac., O.M.D. *Between Heaven and Earth: A Guide to Chinese Medicine.* Ballantine Books, New York; 1991.

Berman BM; Swyers JP Establishing a research agenda for investigating alternative medical interventions for chronic pain. Prim Care 1997 Dec;24(4):743-58

Blalock JE, The Immune System as a Sensory Organ, J.Immunology 1984 Mar 132:3,1067-70.

Burckhardt CS, Clark SR, Bennett RM, Fibromyalgia and quality of life: a comparitive analysis. J. Rheumatol 1993; 20(3): 475-9.

Chaitow, Leon. *The Acupuncture Treatment of Pain.* Healing Arts Press, Rochester, Vermont. 1990.

Chaitow, Leon. *Fibromyalgia and Muscle Pain: What Causes It, How it Feels, and What to Do about It.* Thorsons, SanFrancisco CA, 1995.

Cherniske Stephen. *The DHEA Breakthrough.* Ballantine Books, New York. 1996.

Chopra, Deepak, M.D. *Perfect Health: The Complete Mind/Body Guide.* Harmony Books, New York; 1991.

Chopra, Deepak. *Quantum Healing: Exploring the Frontiers of Mind/Body Medicine,* Bantam Books, New York, 1989.

Croft P, Rigby AS, Boswell R, Schollum J, Silman A. The prevalence of Chronic Widespread Pain in the General Population. Journal of Rheumatology 1993 Apr; 20(4):710-3.

Cunningham ME. Becoming familiar with fibromyalgia. Orthop. Nurs. 15: 33-36 (1996).

Deluze C, Bosia L, Zirbs A, Chantraine A, Vischer TL. Electroacupuncture in fibromyalgia: results of a controlled trial. British Med. J. 1992 Nov 21; 305(6864): 1249-52.

Dilts R, Hallbom T, and Smith S. *Beliefs: Pathways to Health and Well-Being.* Metamorphous Press, Portland Oregon, 1990.

Eden, Donna. *Energy Medicine: Balance Your Body's Energies for Optimum Health, Joy, and vitality,* Tarcher/Putnam Books, New York, 1998.

Elrod, Joe M. *Reversing Fibromyalgia.* Woodland Publishing, Pleasant Grove UT, 1997.

Erickson, MH. *Healing in Hypnosis: The seminars, Workshops, and Lectures of Milton H. Erickson, Vol. 1.* (Ed. EL Rossi, MORyan, FA Sharp). Irvington Publishers Inc. New York 1983.

Gach, Michael Reed. *Acupressure's Potent Points: A Guide to Self-Care for Common Ailments.* Bantam Books, New York 1990.

Goldberg-B. *Alternative medicine guide to chronic fatigue, fibromyalgia & environmental illness.* Future Med Publ (Tiburon, CA) 1998 (359 p)

Goldenberg DI. Fibromyalgia, chronic fatigue syndrome, and myofascial pain. Curr Opin Rhermatol 8: 113-123 (1996).

Goldman JA. Silicone augmentation mammoplasty (SAM): a specific musculoskeletal spectrum due to these implants? Arthritis Rheum 1991; 34: Suppl: R35.

Grady, Harvey. Castor Oil Packs: Scientific Tests Verify Therapeutic Value. Venture Inward; July/August 1988: 12-16.

Granges G, Zilko P, Littlejohn GO. Fibromyalgia Syndrome: Assessment of the Severity of the Condition Two Years after Diagnosis. J. Rheumatol. 1994; 21(3): 523-9.

Greenfield S, Fitzcharies MA, Esdaile JM. Reactive Fibromyalgia Syndrome. Arthritis-Rheum. 1992; 35(6): 678-81.

Gupta S, Vayuvegula B. A comprehensive immunological analysis in chronic fatigue syndrome. Scand. J Immunol 1991 Mar;33(3):319-27.

Haas, Elson M., M.D. *Staying Healthy with the Seasons;* Celestial Arts, Berkeley CA. 1981.

Haas, Elson M. M.D, *Staying Healthy with Nutrition.* Celestial Arts, Berkeley CA, 1992.

Hammer, Leon, M.D. *Dragon Rises, Redbird Flies: Psychology and Chinese Medicine;* Station Hill Press, Barrytown New York, 1990.

Heinerman, John. *Double the Power of Your Immune System,* Parker Publishing, West Nyack New York, 1991.

Higley, Connie and Alan. *Reference Guide for Essential Oils.* Abundant Health Publications, Olath Kansas, 1998.

Hudson J, Goldenberg DD, Pope HG Jr, Keck PE Jr, Schlesinger L. Comorbidity of fibromyalgia with medical and psychiatric disorders. Am. J. Med. 1992; 92(4):363-7.

Kabat-Zinn, J. *Full Catastrophe Living: Using the Wisdom of Your Body and Mind to Face Stress, Pain, and Illness.* Delta Books, New York (1990).

Kapel, P. *The Body Says Yes: Muscle Testing Tunes In to Your Body's Needs.* ACS Publications Inc, San Diego CA 1981.

Kaptchuk, Ted J., O.M.D. *The Web that Has No Weaver- Understanding Chinese Medicine.* Congdon & Weed, New York; 1983.

Kennedy M, Felson DT. A prospective long-term study of fibromyalgia syndrome. Arthritis Rheum 39: 682-685 (1996),

Kobasa SC. Stressful life events, personality, and health: an inquiry into hardiness. J Pers Soc Psychol 1979 Jan;37(1):1-11

Kobasa SC, Maddi SR, Puccetti MC. Personality and exercise as buffers in the stress-illness relationship. J Behav Med 1982 Dec;5(4):391-404

Kobasa SC, Puccetti MC. Personality and social resources in stress resistance. J Pers Soc Psychol 1983 Oct;45(4):839-50

Kobasa SC, Maddi SR, Zola MA. Type A and hardiness. J Behav Med 1983 Mar;6(1):41-51

Kuehn AF, Winters RKV. A study of symptom distress, health locus of control, and coping resources of aging post-polio survivors. Image J. of Nursing Scholarship 1994 Winter 26(4): 325-331.

Lazarou J, Pomeranz BH, Corey PN. Incidence of adverse drug reactions in hospital patients: a meta-analyisis f prospective studies. JAMA, 1998;279:1200-1205.

Ledingham J, Doherty S, Doherty M. Primary Fibromyalgia Syndrome-- an Outcome Study. J. Rheumatol 1993; 32(2):139-42.

Lade, Arnie. *Acupuncture Points: Images and Functions.* Eastland Press, Seattle WA, 1989

Lade, Arnie. *Energetic Healing: Embracing the Life Force.* Lotus Press, Twin Lakes Wisconsin, 1998.

Liberman, Jacob. *Light: Medicine of the Future.* Santa Fe NM: Bear & Co. Publishing, 1991.

Low, Royston. *The Secondary Vessels of Acupuncture.* Thorsons Publishing Group, Northamptonshire England, 1983.

Lu, Henry C. *Chinese System of Food Cures; Prevention and Remedies.* Sterling Publishing Co., New York; 1986.

Maciocia Giovanni. *Tongue Diagnosis in Chinese Medicine.* Eastland Press, Seattle WA; 1987.

Maciocia, Giovanni. *The Foundations of Chinese Medicine: A Comprehensive Text for Acupuncturists and Herbalists.* Churchill Livingstone, New York; 1989

Maciocia G. *The Practice of Chinese Medicine.* Churchill Livingstone, New York 1994.

Mojay, Gabriel. *Aromatherapy for Healing the Spirit.* Owl Books, Henry Holt & Co., New York, 1996.

Myss C, and Shealy CN. *The Creation of Health: The Emotional, Psychological, and Spiritual Responses that Promote Health and Healing.* Three Rivers Press, New York, 1988

Namikoshi, Toru. *The Complete Book of Shiatsu Therapy.* Japan Pub, Tokyo: 1981

Neustaedter R. 1996. Do Vaccines Disable the Immune System?
www.healthy.net/library/articles/neustaedter/immune.htm

Pert CB, "The Wisdom of the Receptors: Neuropeptides, the Emotions, and Bodymind," Advances: Journal of the Institute for the Advancement of Health 3 (3), Summer 1986: 8-16

Peterson C, Semmel A, von Baeyer C, Abramson LY, Metalsky GI, Seligman MEP. 1982. Attributional Style Questionnaire. Cognitive Therapy and Research 6: 287-300.

Pitchford, P. *Healing with Whole Foods: Oriental Traditions and Modern Nutrition.* North Atlantic Books, Berkeley CA. 1993.

Reid, Daniel. *The Complete Book of Chinese Health and Healing.* Shambhala Press, Boston, 1995.

Ritchason J. *The Little Herb Encyclopedia.* Third Edition, Woodland Health Books, Pleasant Grove, UT, 1995.

Ross, Jeremy. *Zang Fu. The Organ Systems of Traditional Chinese Medicine. Functions, Interrelationships, and Patterns of disharmony in Theory and Practice.* Churchill Livingstone, New York 1985.

Rossi, Ernest L. *The Psychobiology of Mind-Body Healing.* W.W. Norton & Co. New York, 1986.

Sanchez-Guerrero J, Colditz GA, Karlson EW, Hunter DJ, Speizer FE, Liang MH. Silicone breast implants and the risk of connective-tissue diseases and symptoms. N Engl J Med 1995; 332: 1666-70.

Seligman MEP, Abramson LY, Semmel A, von Baeyer C. 1979. Depressive attributional style. J. Ab Psych 88:242-247.

Shealy CN, Cady RK, Cox RH, Murrell M. DHEA Deficiency in Patients with Chronic Pain and Depression. J Neurol Orthop Med Surg (1996) 17:6.

Shealy CN. A Review of Dehydroepiandrosterone (DHEA.
Integrative Physiological and Behavioral Science, September-December, 1995. Vol. 30, No. 4, 308-313

Shealy CN, Myss CM. The Ring of Fire and DHEA: A Theory for Energetic Restoration of Adenal Reserves. 1996 Article available online at www.shealyinstitute.com

Smith WA. Fibromyalgia Syndrome. Nursing Clinics of North America 33(4):653-71.

Starlanyl, Devin M.D. and Copeland M.E. *Fibromyalgia and Chronic Myofascial Pain Syndrome: A Survival Manual.* New Harbinger Publications Inc. Oakland CA, 1996.

Taylor ML, Trotter DR Csuka ME. The prevalence of sexual abuse in women with fibromyalgia. Arthritis Rheum. 38: 229-234 (1995)

Teeguarden, Iona Marsaa, M.A., M.F.C.C. *Joy of Feeling: Bodymind Acupressure.* Japan Publications Inc., Tokyo and New York; 1984.

Teitelbaum, Jacob M.D. *From Fatigued to Fantastic: A Manual for moving beyond chronic fatigue and fibromyalgia.* Deva Press, Annapolis MD 1995.

Tierra M. *Planetary Herbology.* Lotus Press, Santa Fe NM. 1988.

Temoshok L, Dreher H. *The Type C Connection. The Behavioral Links to Cancer and Your Health.* Random House, New York; 1992.

Van Why, RP. Fibromyalgia Syndrome and Massage Therapy: Issues and Opportunitie.. 1998 . Contains extensive bibliiography of medical literature on fibromyalgia syndrome. Order from author 123 E 8th St, #121, Frederick MD 21701

Vasey FB, Havice DL, Bocanegra TS, et al. Clinical findings in symptomatic women with silicone breast implants. Semin Arthritis Rheum 1994;24: Suppl 1:22-8.

VonViczay M. Move Your Lymph. Alternative Medicine Digest, Issue 9 (1996): 22-24.

Waylonis GW, Heck W, Fibromyalgia Syndrome: New Associations. Am. J. Phys. Med. Rehabil. 1992; 71(6):343-8.

Weibel RE, Benor DE. Chronic arthropathy and musculoskeletal symptoms associated with rubella vaccines. A review of 124 claims submitted to the National Vaccine Injury Compensation Program. Arthritis Rheum, 1996 Sep, 39:9, 1529-34

Wiedenfeld SA, O'Leary A, Bandura A, Brown S, Levine S, Raska K, Impact of perceived self-efficacy in coping with stressors on components of the immune system. J Pers Soc Psychol 1990 Nov;59(5):1082-94

Young A. Amma Therapy, A holistic approach to chronic fatigue syndrome. J. Holistic Nurs. 1993 June ; 2(2): 172-182.

Zhen Li Shi , *Pulse Diagnosis.* Translated by Hoc Ku Huynh, Edited by G.M. Siefert; Paradigm Publications, Brookline Mass; 1981.

Zi, Nancy. *The Art of Breathing: Thirty Simple Exercises for Improving your Performance and Well-Being.* Bantam, San Francisco, 1986.

INDEX

QUICK AND EASY ORDER FORM

TELL A COLLEAGUE OR FRIEND ABOUT THIS BOOK, OR GIVE AS A GIFT!

TELEPHONE ORDERS: Call (801)-612-1306. Books will be shipped and billed when order is received.

E-MAIL ORDERS: ShuPoint@aol.com. Books will be shipped and billed when order is received

POSTAL MAIL ORDERS: Life Circles Publications, 965 East 28th Street, Ogden UT 84403. Telephone (801)-612-1306.

Please send the following books:
_____ Copies of *"Fibromyalgia and Chronic Fatigue Syndrome: Acutherapy and Holistic Approaches."* (Retail price $27.95)

Please send FREE information on:

_____ Upcoming Book "Traditional Chinese Medical Theory"
_____ Seminars and Workshops on Chinese Medicine, Bodywork, Holistic Health; Massage and Bodywork CEU Trainings

Your Name or Company_____
Shipping Address _____
City, State, Zip _____
Telephone _____ Email _____
Billing Address (if different from shipping address)
_____ _ _

Sales Tax: Please add 6.25% to products shipped to Utah addresses.

Shipping: Multiple-copy orders will be sent by ground UPS or US Postal Book rate, whichever is less. Single copies will be sent US PRIORITY mail, $3.20 per book. Purchaser pays shipping/postage charges.

For single-book orders, refer to the table below for amounts.

	US orders Outside Utah	Utah Addresses
Single copy:	$27.95	$27.95
Priority Mail	$3.20	$3.20
Sales Tax	-------	$1.75
Totals	$31.15	$32.90

For discount rates and terms and conditions for multiple-copy orders for resale, call, Email, or write to Life Circles Publications.

THANK YOU FOR YOUR ORDER!
LIFE CIRCLES PUBLICATIONS

QUICK AND EASY ORDER FORM

TELL A COLLEAGUE OR FRIEND ABOUT THIS BOOK, OR GIVE AS A GIFT!

TELEPHONE ORDERS: Call (801)-612-1306. Books will be shipped and billed when order is received.

E-MAIL ORDERS: ShuPoint@aol.com. Books will be shipped and billed when order is received

POSTAL MAIL ORDERS: Life Circles Publications, 965 East 28th Street, Ogden UT 84403. Telephone (801)-612-1306.

Please send the following books:
_____ Copies of *"Fibromyalgia and Chronic Fatigue Syndrome: Acutherapy and Holistic Approaches."* (Retail price $27.95)

Please send FREE information on:

_____ Upcoming Book "Traditional Chinese Medical Theory"
_____ Seminars and Workshops on Chinese Medicine, Bodywork, Holistic Health; Massage and Bodywork CEU Trainings

Your Name or Company_____
Shipping Address _____
City, State, Zip _____
Telephone _____ Email _____
Billing Address (if different from shipping address)

_____ __ __

Sales Tax: Please add 6.25% to products shipped to Utah addresses.

Shipping: Multiple-copy orders will be sent by ground UPS or US Postal Book rate, whichever is less. Single copies will be sent US PRIORITY mail, $3.20 per book. Purchaser pays shipping/postage charges.

For single-book orders, refer to the table below for amounts.

	US orders Outside Utah	Utah Addresses
Single copy:	$27.95	$27.95
Priority Mail	$3.20	$3.20
Sales Tax	-------	$1.75
Totals	$31.15	$32.90

For discount rates and terms and conditions for multiple-copy orders for resale, call, Email, or write to Life Circles Publications.

THANK YOU FOR YOUR ORDER!
LIFE CIRCLES PUBLICATIONS